DIAGNOSIS FEMALE

DIAGNOSIS FEMALE

How Medical Bias Endangers Women's Health

Emily Dwass

ROWMAN & LITTLEFIELD
Lanham • Boulder • New York • London

Published by Rowman & Littlefield
An imprint of The Rowman & Littlefield Publishing Group, Inc.
4501 Forbes Boulevard, Suite 200, Lanham, Maryland 20706
www.rowman.com

86-90 Paul Street, London EC2A 4NE, United Kingdom

British Library Cataloguing in Publication Information Available

Library of Congress Cataloging-in-Publication Data

Names: Dwass, Emily, 1953– author.
Title: Diagnosis female : how medical bias endangers women's health / Emily Dwass.
Description: Lanham : Rowman & Littlefield, 2019. | Includes bibliographical references and index.
Identifiers: LCCN 2019005447 (print) | LCCN 2019014125 (ebook) | ISBN 9781538114476 (elec-
    tronic) | ISBN 9781538114469 (cloth : alk. paper) | ISBN 9781538164716 (pbk. : alk. paper)
Subjects: LCSH: Women—Health and hygiene—Sociological aspects. | Women—Diseases. | Wom-
    en's health services—Social aspects.
Classification: LCC RA564.85 (ebook) | LCC RA564.85 .D92 2019 (print) | DDC 613/.04244—dc23
LC record available at https://lccn.loc.gov/2019005447

To my wonderful family,
who give me symptoms of joy every day

CONTENTS

INTRODUCTION

When I was growing up in suburban Chicago, our pediatrician was a kind man who made house calls, sometimes twice in one day. No matter what was wrong with me or my three siblings, he had the cure, instilling the idea that doctors would always have an answer. That assumption was upended when I was an undergraduate at the University of Illinois and went to the student health service for help with severe menstrual cramps. A young female doctor folded her arms and looked askance before declaring: "Some women get cramps because they don't like having periods." And that was the extent of her exam, diagnosis, and treatment.

I figured that this unhelpful appointment was due to the nature of student healthcare in the 1970s. (One of my roommates went to the same medical center with a urinary tract infection and was given a morality lecture instead of antibiotics.) But in the years after college, unsettling doctor appointments continued. They ranged from condescending (a rheumatologist who started things off by asking, "What's your story of woe?") to dangerous (a brain tumor that was misdiagnosed for four years).

I was hardly alone. In researching this book, I found a theme that reverberated in the stories of the women who shared their medical journeys with me—time and again, they said that their voices did not matter, or worse, that their concerns were dismissed when they sought help for medical problems. Not only were they greeted with skepticism when they described their symptoms, but they also encountered an astounding lack of empathy.

Critical care physician Dr. Rana Awdish, director of the Pulmonary Hypertension Program at Henry Ford Hospital in Detroit—who barely survived a catastrophic medical crisis during her first pregnancy—told me that she believes "women are more vulnerable in every dynamic. I think that in so many ways we've been taught to invalidate our own truth and only know things about ourselves when we're told them. That cultural bias of devaluing our own experience translates into medicine as well." (*Note*: In this book, quotations without citations are from interviews with the author. Quotes with other origins have footnotes indicating the source.)

Some of the problems that women encounter in their healthcare are rooted in labs, where for generations scientific research was strictly a boys' club. And I'm not just referring to the scientists looking into microscopes. For most of medical history, all of the cells, tissues, animals, and people being studied were male. Unbelievably, women were excluded as medical research subjects until 1993, meaning that most of what is now known about drugs and diseases is based on findings applicable to only half the population.

There's no question that the exclusion of women from scientific research seeped into clinical practice. Deeply ingrained in both areas of medicine was the belief that men and women were basically the same, with the exception of the "bikini zone." This meant that doctors expected female symptoms to look like male symptoms. If women presented differently, all too often the diagnosis was some version of "all in her head." This has had dire consequences for women seeking medical care. Take, for example, heart attacks. Chest pain and pressure are the unmistakable signs of cardiac distress—in men. A woman, on the other hand, may exhibit extreme fatigue as her primary symptom. Doctors who are unaware of this won't think to investigate further, putting the patient at risk.

You can draw a straight line from faulty research conclusions—based on scientific studies that ignored women—to mistakes in medical settings. Even when it finally became accepted that, biologically, women were not mini-men, many clinicians did not get the memo. "We aren't even close to closing the gap of knowledge on women's health. To this day, we are utilizing evidence that is based upon research that was done on men," said Dr. Alyson J. McGregor, director of the Division of Sex and Gender in Emergency Medicine at Brown University.

She continued: "When people use the words 'gender bias,' I'm always a little hesitant, because it's not necessarily a conscious bias, although that still exists in every element of our society. When you think about what's happening when a physician is seeing a patient and that patient is describing their symptoms, all of the medical knowledge that that physician is using has been based on research done on men. The bias is there in the knowledge of how the human body responds. It's ingrained into the diagnostic testing choices that we have. When we order a test, that test was affected and designed to detect the way that men have a disease. If a woman comes in, her symptoms may not be exactly what we're expecting, because we're expecting the symptoms of certain things that have occurred in men. And then the physician—whether they're male or female, it doesn't matter—will they even recognize that particular symptom as something that is concerning?"

Dr. McGregor, coauthor of the medical textbook *Sex and Gender in Acute Medical Care*, explained that an ongoing risk for women is that doctors view male patterns of disease as typical and female patterns as atypical. In fact, with the same condition, there can be specific symptoms that are common in men and others that are the norm for women. "By viewing women and their presentations as *atypical*, it leads to this lack of recognition that women may have different ramifications of the same illness. . . . That's a very serious issue when women seek emergency care," said Dr. McGregor.

She noted that even when a correct diagnosis is made, there is the question of whether or not the treatment plan is known to be effective for women: "When we prescribe medication to women, it can be a guessing game as to what that medication will do, whether it's a high enough dose, a low enough dose, and what the side effects may be. These concerns are ingrained into the entire medical system."

It is only in recent years that scientists have realized that studies done solely on male cells, male animals, or human males can have a domino effect in disease management and in medication. For example, in 2013 the Food and Drug Administration (FDA) recommended that the dosage of the sleeping pill Zolpidem (sold under different brand names, including Ambien) be lowered by half for women after it was discovered that the original dosing instructions were more likely to leave women with next-day impairment. Because men and women metabolize the sleeping medication differently, the same dose could leave a woman with the drug still in her body the next morning, affecting her ability to safely drive.[1]

The US Government Accountability Office reported that eight of the ten prescription drugs withdrawn from the market between 1997 and 2001 were shown to pose greater health risks for women than for men.[2] As reported in the *New York Times*, "Sleeping pills are hardly the only medications that may have unexpected, even dangerous, effects in women. Studies have shown that women respond differently than men to many drugs, from aspirin to anesthesia."[3]

The Zolpidem saga drove home the point that drug researchers need to investigate the different ways men and women may respond to medications. Biochemist Nicole Woitowich, PhD, associate director of the Women's Health Research Institute at Northwestern University, said the lessons learned from Zolpidem were huge. "When we try to explain to people who are not as familiar with scientific research about how it is important to consider sex as a biological variable—sometimes these words can get lost and misconstrued," explained Dr. Woitowich. "But when you say that there was a drug that was developed and women and men were both taking it, but women were having these adverse effects, that paints a much clearer picture."

Females have been excluded even from studies of conditions that primarily affect women. Depression is known to be a major cause of disability in women across the globe. Yet the majority of brain research has been done exclusively on male animals.[4] It's no surprise, then, that women may respond differently to antidepressants. While women are twice as likely to be given a prescription for a psychotropic medication, they are more apt to experience unpleasant or dangerous side effects. With anti-anxiety meds, due to acidity levels in their stomachs, women may absorb the drugs faster, and the prescribed dose may be more toxic.[5]

Another striking example is the research that has been done on Rett syndrome, a rare, genetically based neurological disorder that strikes infants, causing devastating disability. Nearly all of the affected individuals are girls. But for decades, most of the research on the disorder was done on male animals.[6]

And in yet another "*Huh?*" moment, for a small study of the first-ever female libido pill, Addyi, there were twenty-five participants—and twenty-three of them were men. The FDA approved this medication in 2015 as a treatment for female sexual dysfunction based on research done on "a population of 92 percent men for a drug intended only for women."[7]

If these were isolated scientific missteps, we could view them simply as blips in the medical landscape. But rather than being deviations from common practice, they have been the routine in studies done on diseases and drugs. The underrepresentation of women in scientific research echoes women's exclusion in other parts of society, with one big difference: It endangers women's health.

"When we think about gender bias, we have to go back in history to when there was this misperception that men and women were the same biologically, except for reproductive organs—our brains, our hearts, our lungs were thought to be no different. This went on for hundreds if not thousands of years," says Dr. Marjorie Jenkins, an internist at Texas Tech University Health Sciences Center and the founding director and chief scientific officer of the Laura W. Bush Institute for Women's Health. Government policies categorized women as a group that needed protection, along with children, the elderly, and prisoners. Even if a woman of reproductive age gave informed consent and said that she wanted to join in clinical trials of new medication, she was prohibited from participating.

Awareness that women's health was being harmed by research exclusion began to emerge in the 1960s and 1970s, with different lay groups sounding the alarm. This movement came on the heels of three healthcare catastrophes: birth defects caused by the sedative thalidomide; the deadly Dalkon Shield intrauterine device; and the drug diethylstilbestrol, which was given to pregnant women to prevent miscarriages (despite research showing the drug didn't work) and which subsequently caused vaginal cancer in many of the daughters of women who took it. These tragedies led to the 1977 FDA recommendation that women of reproductive age be excluded from early phase studies of drug testing, except in cases of life-threatening illnesses.[8]

Early advocates were inspired when the Boston Women's Health Book Collective published a booklet in 1970, which evolved into the pioneering bestseller *Our Bodies, Ourselves*. At the same time, as more women were attending medical school, awareness grew about inequities in healthcare, with major studies driving home the point that women were being ignored. The Baltimore Longitudinal Study of Aging was launched by the National Institutes of Health (NIH) in 1958 with seventy-five thousand male participants. Observed US Representative Patricia Schroeder (D-CO), who served from 1972 to 1996: "The study did not address osteoporosis, bladder incontinence, menopause and other age-related issues of particular concern to women. We asked why women were not part of the study since women have a longer life expectancy than men and constitute a higher percentage of the aging population. NIH told us it was easier for research subjects to use the men's restrooms at their facilities."[9] (Women joined the study in 1978.)[10]

In 1980, scientists began research to find out if taking low-dose aspirin could reduce the risk of heart attack. It was the largest study of its kind, with 22,071 participants—and nary one female.[11] The researchers were operating under the long-ingrained and erroneous assumption that heart disease was a male problem. (In fact, cardiovascular disease and stroke cause one in three women's deaths each year, killing a woman every eighty seconds.)[12] Another major study, which ran from 1972 to 1998, examined the role of exercise and diet in preventing heart disease. The Multiple Risk Factor Intervention Trial (MRFIT) had thirteen thousand male participants and, again, zero women.

Dr. Ruth Kirschstein—who made history in 1974 by becoming the first female institute director at the NIH, as well as for her work in developing safer vaccines—spoke out about the link between lack of research on women's health issues and threats to the medical care they receive. In 1985 she launched a Public Health Service task force report, which prompted the NIH to suggest that studies using federal research funds should include women. The report, which came out in 1986, recommended that biomedical and behavioral research be expanded to assure "appropriate emphasis" on conditions and diseases that strike women of all ages.[13]

On paper, this sounded like progress for women's health. In reality, most researchers ignored the policy recommendation. In 1991 cardiologist Dr. Bernadine Healy became the first female director of the NIH. She launched the NIH Women's Health Initiative, a $500 million campaign to study health conditions that affect women.[14] A breakthrough came with the implementation of the 1993 NIH Revitalization Act and its mandate to include women in research trials funded by the government. The legislation also called for the inclusion of racial minorities, another group that had long been neglected in scientific studies.[15]

Looking back at the important changes in medical research over the years, ophthalmologist Dr. Janine Austin Clayton, who was appointed director of the NIH Office of Research on Women's Health in 2012, reflected on barriers to women's inclusion, including protectionism, paternalism, and concerns that women's variable hormonal status could not be adequately controlled.[16]

In a 2018 *Forbes* profile, Dr. Clayton talked about the disturbing gender disparities that still exist in medical research and care: "As a woman myself, I'd like to know that any treatment that is being recommended for me has been tested in women and men. . . . If we do not take into consideration what I feel is the most important fundamental biological variable—being male or female—we run the risk of making errors in our [medical] conclusions."[17]

The terms *sex* and *gender* are often used interchangeably, but they have different meanings in medical research: In science, *sex* refers to specific biological traits, based on genetic makeup. *Gender* is how we see and present ourselves in society—socially, culturally, and sexually. (The current government has a different view of sex and gender, and as I write this, the Trump administration is seeking to roll back the federal civil rights of transgender individuals by "narrowly defining gender as a biological, immutable condition determined by genitalia at birth."[18])

Both sex and gender can influence our health, and there can be bias on both fronts. Our sex can have a profound impact on the diseases we get, how these diseases manifest, and how they respond to treatments. Gender can affect how we are viewed and how we are treated—or sometimes mistreated—when we are in need of medical care.[19]

"One's sex impacts one's health in many ways," said Kathryn Sandberg, PhD, director of the Center for the Study of Sex Differences at Georgetown University in Washington, DC, who has been a leading advocate for the inclusion of sex as a biological variable in medical research. She explained that to truly understand the cause, development, and pathology of diseases, the sex of study participants must be taken into account, especially in the growing realm of personalized medicine. This kind of research benefits both men and women and is key to answering questions such as: Why are men more prone to certain viral infections? Why do women tend to get a form of lung cancer that is tougher to treat? Why are men more likely to die from tuberculosis? Why are 75 percent of people who have autoimmune diseases women? "While males and females may be included in studies, if they don't analyze the data by sex, then what's the point?" asked Dr. Sandberg.

A 2001 Institute of Medicine report noted that despite progress that has been made, research has limited value unless sex (being biologically male or female) is recognized as a key variable.[20] The report pointed out while it is anatomically obvious why only men get prostate cancer and only women get ovarian cancer, it is not obvious why females are more likely than males to recover language ability after suffering a left-hemisphere stroke or why females have a greater risk than males of developing life-threatening heart problems from certain drugs.[21]

"Men and women are different down to the cellular and molecular levels. It means that we're different across all of our organs, from our brains, our hearts, our lungs, our joints," said cardiologist Dr. Paula Johnson, president of Wellesley College, in a 2017 TED Talk, pointing out that every cell has a sex.[22]

Larry Cahill, PhD, a neuroscientist at the University of California, Irvine, explained to correspondent Lesley Stahl on *60 Minutes* why it's not enough for researchers to simply add women and mix: "If you're clumping men and women together in your study and there truly is a sex difference, you're not just harming the women; you're harming the men. You're muddling up the understanding of what's going on, you're muddling up the path to clear treatment."[23]

Texas Tech's Dr. Jenkins pointed out that bringing more awareness to gender bias in healthcare helps all patients: "There is still this underlying tendency for the health care professions to *sex* diseases: So women get depression, men get heart disease. Women get osteoporosis, and men get COPD or emphysema. That's inherently biased, because, for example, men are more likely to die from osteoporosis when they break a bone. Men with osteoporosis are underdiagnosed; they're underscreened. The gender lens goes both ways."

One of the goals of Northwestern University's Women's Health Research Institute is to educate and assist researchers, in order to enable them to conduct sex-based or sex-inclusive research, said Dr. Woitowich. "I've asked trainees, 'Do you know the sex of your cells?' And they responded, 'Oh, I've never thought about that.' There is a lack of awareness about the influence of sex in basic science research, and that's why we provide education and training so that sex will be considered in the same way as the other variables in an experiment."

Twenty years after the 1993 congressional mandate ordering the NIH to include women in biomedical research, a report by George Washington University in Washington, DC, and Brigham and Women's Hospital in Boston found that women continued to face health risks because their medical treatments are based on studies that left out females or did not break down the results to determine how women might be affected. The study authors noted that this deficit in research is ongoing, while rates of lung cancer, heart disease, Alzheimer's, and depression are on the rise among women.[24]

In 2013 Georgetown University's Dr. Sandberg and Scott Fleming, then the school's associate vice president for federal relations, asked Rep. Nita Lowey of New York and Rep. Rosa DeLauro of Connecticut to push for a mandate that federally funded scientific research must include female cells and female animals. (Both representatives had been instrumental in the passage of the 1993 NIH Revitalization Act.)

Pushed on by Dr. Sandberg and Mr. Fleming, the two politicians wrote to NIH director Dr. Francis Collins, who responded with a commentary in the May 2014 journal *Nature* in which he and Dr. Clayton pledged to improve the balance of male and female subjects in preclinical research supported by NIH.[25]

In January 2016 NIH began requiring all applications for research funding to account for the possible role of sex as a biological variable in vertebrate animal and human studies. UC Irvine's Dr. Cahill describes this action as "historic, because it was in essence a corner turned that cannot be unturned," requiring researchers to consider the differences between males and females "or give us a damn good reason why not. Those are your choices. There's no more dismissing it and trivializing it and explaining it away."

Dr. Cahill has been an important force in the movement to change how medical research is conducted. He initially became aware of this cause by accident, in 2000, when he was conducting studies in his lab on emotional memory. While looking at the amygdala, a part of the brain involved with how emotions are experienced, he found distinct differences between males and females. "That became a fork in the road that changed my whole scientific life," he told me, leading him to wonder: "Is Mother Nature trying to tell me something here? What if we have had blinders on? What if there are sex influences all over the place that we've missed in animal research because we just study the male?"

When he decided to devote his career to pursuing this line of inquiry, senior colleagues tried to dissuade him from studying sex and gender differences in medical research, warning him that this was a waste of time and could even turn him into an academic pariah. The message he received was that there was no way attitudes and practices in medicine were going to change. "Between 2000 and 2016 sometimes you just felt like you were spitting into a hurricane," observed Dr. Cahill.

Georgetown's Dr. Sandberg pointed out that while the landmark 2016 NIH requirement was a big step in the right direction, it is not safe to assume that the research requirement is always being followed. One of the areas of study in her lab is renal dysfunction associated with hypertension. Shortly before we talked, she looked at all of the recent animal studies on this topic, which had been published in top journals. "I looked at how many were conducted just on males, how many were conducted just on females, and how many were conducted on males and females. In one journal it was five to one, males to females. In another, it was eleven to one, males to females and in the other it was sixteen to one, males to females. Terrible! And that was in 2017, *after* NIH had put this rule into effect," Dr. Sandberg said.

One of the biggest remaining hurdles is that it's often impossible to know the sex of research subjects because it has not been reported, said Dr. Woitowich: "As scientists, if we don't know what other researchers are doing, or if they've been testing males, females, or both sexes, it's hard for us to recapitulate those studies. There's a whole body of knowledge that we're missing. . . . This is not the best way to conduct science, plain and simple."

A tangential concern with medical studies is the lack of transparency about researchers' financial ties to the drug and medical device industries, which may end up skewing results and ultimately affecting treatments that make their way to patients. A 2018 investigation by ProPublica and the *New York Times* revealed that Dr. José Baselga, a renowned breast cancer researcher and the chief medical officer at Memorial Sloan Kettering Cancer Center in New York, failed to disclose his financial conflicts of interests in studies that affected breast cancer treatments. The investigation led to Dr. Baselga's resignation, as well as urgent questions about how medical research is influenced by industry ties. As the journalists investigating the problem noted: "Ethicists worry that outside entangle-ments can shape the way studies are designed and medications are pre-scribed to patients, allowing bias to influence medical practice. Disclos-ing those connections allows the public, other scientists and doctors to evaluate the research and weigh potential conflicts."[26]

The 2018 documentary *The Bleeding Edge* brings to light inadequate-ly tested and poorly monitored medical devices that sicken both men and women, while exposing how doctors are vulnerable to industry incentives to promote new surgical tools. The film showcases women who have suffered horrific disability from Johnson & Johnson's pelvic mesh, used to treat urinary leakage and pelvic organ prolapse; Bayer's Essure birth control implant (removed from the market when the movie was released); and Intuitive Surgical's da Vinci Surgical System, a robotic surgery sys-tem that maimed women during hysterectomies.[27]

One of the documentary's producers and writers, Amy Ziering, told me that women are particularly at risk from medical devices because many tools brought to market were tested on male subjects. She added that while medical devices can be lifesaving, "the chase for profits should not trump patient safety, and unfortunately, all too often it does."

Now living with chronic pain and poor health, the women featured in the film learned that the doctors who had so eagerly promoted these supposed medical innovations had neither compassion nor solutions when the devices caused permanent harm.[28] And once a woman is living with ongoing pain, getting help is not easy. In her article "Gender Bias and the Ongoing Need to Acknowledge Women's Pain," Amy M. Miller, PhD, president and CEO of the Society for Women's Health Research, pointed out that nearly 80 percent of animal studies published in the journal *Pain* from 1996 to 2005 used male subjects: "With society often dismissing women's pain and a relatively brief record of research inclusive of wom-en, it is unsurprising that many of the chronic pain conditions for which we do not have direct treatments are more common in or exclusively affect women."[29]

The devastating opioid crisis is complicated by a lack of understand-ing of pain in women and how women respond to opioids, said orthopedic surgeon Dr. Kimberly Templeton, a professor at the University of Kansas Medical Center. She has been trying to raise awareness that despite the focus on the opioid crisis, there is not a lot of discussion about how pain is different in men and women. Not only are women more likely to have conditions that lead to chronic pain, they may have a different perception of pain, based on how their spinal cords and brains process pain signals. In addition, women's chronic pain may be more severe due to coexisting depression or post-traumatic stress, and some women may be self-medicating with opioids. "Currently, the group that has the highest rate of increase in opioid-related deaths is middle-aged women. That's a group that has not received much attention. Like every other health condition, there are sex- and gender-related differences in pain and response to opioids," said Dr. Templeton, a former president of the United States Bone and Joint Initiative and the American Medical Women's Association (AMWA).

Or consider the status of knees. Over the course of a lifetime, nearly half of American adults will develop osteoarthritis in at least one knee, but women typically are significantly more disabled before being referred to an orthopedic surgeon. Not only can knee pain be debilitating, it contributes to other medical problems. "It's concerning when people say it's 'just' joint pain," said Dr. Templeton. "No, it's not *just* joint pain. There is the impact of joint pain on your quality of life, and also on many of the other health conditions that you may have"—for example, not being able to exercise because your knees hurt can make you gain weight, which makes your knees hurt more, leading to a vicious cycle. Joint pain also can make it more difficult to use exercise as part of the treatment regimen for heart disease and diabetes.

Texas Tech's Dr. Jenkins pointed out that women are twenty-five times less likely than men to be referred for knee replacement surgery, with the same amount of arthritis and the same amount of pain. "That's not a sex difference, that is gender bias," said Dr. Jenkins. In that scenario, with a doctor dismissing symptoms, some women become reluctant to advocate for themselves. And if a physician does not acknowledge their pain, they may conclude that their own discomfort is not important. The landmark paper "The Girl Who Cried Pain: A Bias against Women in the Treatment of Pain" noted a large body of evidence that women are less likely to receive effective treatment, with some being prescribed sedatives instead of pain medication.[30]

Such skepticism, bias, and undertreatment are echoed in other areas of medicine as well. In her book about treating patients with Alzheimer's disease (nearly two-thirds of Americans with Alzheimer's are women),[31] neurologist Dr. Gayatri Devi wrote about the sad diagnosis she gave to

Rosa, the sister of a patient who had died of an aggressive form of the disease. Dr. Devi suspected that Rosa was suffering from the same hopeless form of dementia. When she was invited to present a case during grand rounds, she brought in Rosa, hoping that the renowned neurologist leading the session might offer fresh insights. After examining the patient, the neurologist gave his diagnosis: Rosa was hysterical and making up symptoms in order to receive disability benefits. He also concluded that Rosa was "malingering for secondary gain." Dr. Devi was aghast.[32]

She reflected on the experience: "I was beyond angry. The malingering part was particularly insulting, implying as it did that Rosa was faking her symptoms. At least the hysteria part of his diagnosis, although also insulting, implied that there was an unconscious psychological cause of her symptoms, albeit with a clear gender bias. Hysteria is a term coined in 1900 BC—almost 4,000 years ago—to describe inexplicable symptoms in women. It still exists as a diagnosis in the clinical lexicon, but is rarely found in textbooks anymore. . . . Rosa was not alone in being misdiagnosed like this, although her story is the most egregious I've encountered. Too often women get dismissed, their complaints labeled as 'hysteria' or written off as anxiety. . . . [A] new generation of medical students and some of the neurologists in the auditorium that day will have this ludicrous diagnosis spring to mind when they see a woman with symptoms similar to Rosa."[33]

When a doctor shrugs off or incorrectly analyzes symptoms, a process is set in motion that can result in misdiagnosis and delayed treatment, sometimes with catastrophic results. It's a widespread problem that affects women of all ages and walks of life. Even the powerful and revered are not immune. In a *Wall Street Journal* profile Oprah Winfrey talked about a health crisis she went through in her fifties, when a thyroid condition was not diagnosed in a timely manner: "I thought I was dying every night, because I had heart palpitations. I went to five different doctors, and each of them gave me a prescription for a different kind of heart medication, and it turned out I didn't have a heart problem at all."[34]

Most Americans, both men and women, will have to deal with a medical misdiagnosis at some point in their lives. Experts say that one in twenty adults experiences a diagnostic or treatment error each year. Dr. Robert Pearl, former chief executive of Kaiser Permanente, wrote in an op-ed that many mistakes can be avoided, some by common sense, such as "insisting all medical staff wash their hands between patient visits.

Studies show that they don't a third of the time, which can allow transmission of deadly infections from one person to the next."[35] A study by Johns Hopkins University calculated that more than 250,000 US patient deaths annually are due to medical error.[36]

This statistic is frightening for everyone—but women have extra reason to be worried, because they frequently face the extra burden of not having their symptoms believed. For a woman with autoimmune symptoms, this may result in going to multiple doctors for years before someone takes the time to really investigate what is going on. For a woman with neurological symptoms it might mean being sent for a psychological evaluation before having a brain scan. For a woman experiencing a stroke it might mean being told she has a migraine.

"When a woman walks into a medical office, as compared to a man, the doctor, depending on how the doctor is attuned to his or her own biases, may perceive that the woman doesn't really have a serious disease," said endocrinologist Dr. Connie Newman, an adjunct professor at New York University School of Medicine and the 2017–2018 president of AMWA. "Sometimes the doctor thinks that her symptoms are psychologically derived. That's what we mean by gender bias in medical care: expectations due to attitudes that the healthcare provider has because of the gender of the patient, whether that patient is a woman or a man. Doctors may feel differently when they see women and when they see men. And these biases are hard for doctors to recognize. I think we have a long way to go."

While older women sometimes experience gender bias as well as ageism, younger women may face different challenges. Dr. Sami Saba, a neurologist at Lenox Hill Hospital in New York City, told me that a lack of awareness among doctors contributes to misdiagnoses of young women, because that patient population is expected to be healthy. Dr. Saba said that when a young woman seeks help for unusual symptoms, a physician may think: "'You're twenty-five; look at you, you're in good shape.' The doctor concludes that the patient doesn't look sick, so she can't be sick—not realizing that a lot of diseases, like multiple sclerosis and migraines, can start in women who are in their twenties."

In a letter to the editor in the *New Yorker*, Dr. Saba wrote that women—especially women of color—"are often disbelieved and dismissed by medical professionals. This is indeed an immense problem. I have given diagnoses of neurological illnesses to many women who had previously been told—often by multiple physicians—that their symptoms were merely psychological."[37]

Even the most conscientious of doctors sometimes are swayed by implicit bias. "We like to think that we're not biased, but everyone's biased in a certain way. Being aware of the bias and trying to overcome that is important. That's something that's very hard for people to do," said Dr. Saba. "I can think of a few cases in which I caught myself being prejudiced and wanted to do a better job the next time." He explained that when he was in residency, he worked at Bellevue Hospital in New York City, where he treated inmates from Rikers Island. He had heard that prisoners sometimes faked symptoms in order to get away from a dangerous situation in jail. "Going through your training there, it's easy to dismiss the prisoners' complaints," said Dr. Saba. "There was a case where I sent a guy back from the ER to Rikers, saying that there's nothing wrong with him. And he came back the next week and he had multiple sclerosis. He was having a bad flare, and he had no previous diagnosis of multiple sclerosis. I felt terrible about that. I thought, 'From now on, I'm going to be more careful about these prisoners.' Because they're disadvantaged, my bar should be even higher for the care that I give them."

Gender bias in medical care can start at a young age, having long-term repercussions. For example, autism spectrum disorders in girls often go unrecognized and are underdiagnosed at key developmental points, meaning girls are missing out on life-changing interventions. One explanation—again—is that the criteria used to diagnose autism is based on research that was done almost exclusively on boys.[38]

Women navigating the maze of medical care sometimes encounter unexpected bias. Journalist Alanna Weissman wrote about the five years she spent trying to have a permanent procedure to make sure she would never get pregnant; doctor after doctor second-guessed her decision to remain childless. She was dismayed that even in "deep-blue New York City I was met by doctors who, it seemed, thought they knew me better than I knew myself."[39]

It's no shock that bias against women exists on the internet, but it is surprising that it shows up on Wikipedia. Katherine Maher, executive director of the foundation that runs the website, wrote an op-ed about how Wikipedia underrepresents the accomplishments of women in science and medicine: "Wikipedia articles about health get close attention from our community of medical editors, but for years, some articles on critical women's health issues, such as breastfeeding, languished under a 'low importance' categorization. . . . Increasingly, Wikipedia's content and any biases therein have ramifications well beyond our own website."[40]

Bias that endangers women's health can happen in the White House, in Congress, on the Supreme Court, and even in neighborhood pharmacies. In 2018 a CVS pharmacist in Arizona refused to fill a hormone prescription for Hilde Hall, a transgender woman; he loudly questioned her in front of other customers, then would not return her prescription slip, so she could take it to another pharmacy. Hilde wrote that the encounter left her "embarrassed and stressed. . . . I felt like the pharmacist was trying to out me as transgender in front of strangers. . . . My family supports me, fortunately, and helped me work through the anger and humiliation this experience caused. But many other transgender people are not as fortunate as I am. I don't want to think about what might happen if this pharmacist mistreats a transgender person who does not have a good social support system."[41] (CVS ended up firing the pharmacist.)

In another disturbing incident, a Walgreen's pharmacist in Arizona refused to fill Nicole Arteaga's prescription after she received the heart-breaking news that her pregnancy was not viable. She tried to explain her tragic situation to the pharmacist, telling him that her options to end the pregnancy were to take medication or to have surgery. But the pharmacist still would not serve her.[42] Under Arizona law, pharmacists are within their legal rights to refuse to fill prescriptions, even though this goes against the profession's Oath of a Pharmacist, which includes the mandate to "respect and protect all personal and health information entrusted to me."[43]

Gender bias of a different sort comes into play when the government tries to control women's reproductive health. This has filtered into political stances. On March 30, 2016, candidate Donald Trump told MSNBC's Chris Matthews that "there has to be some form of punishment" for women who have abortions. When Mr. Matthews asked, "What about the guy who gets her pregnant?"—should he also be punished? Mr. Trump replied, "I would say, 'no.'"[44]

If the idea of punishing pregnant women in the United States sounds far-fetched, it is, in fact, already a reality. Lynn M. Paltrow, founder and executive director of National Advocates for Pregnant Women, wrote that her organization has documented some twelve hundred cases of pregnant women being arrested or detained for endangering their unborn baby, because they "fell down a flight of stairs, delayed having cesarean surgery, had a home birth, used a controlled substance (including ones prescribed to them), experienced miscarriages and stillbirths or who gave birth to a baby who did not survive. Such arrests have occurred in virtually every state, including New York, which is one of the eight states that has a law specifically making self-abortion a crime."[45]

In writing about the hazards pregnant women may face, author Kim Brooks told the story of Thea, who was at her final prenatal appointment when her doctor told her she needed to be induced immediately. When Thea asked if she could go get her overnight bag, the doctor told her if she left the premises she could be arrested for putting her child in danger.[46] Indiana resident Purvi Patel was sentenced to twenty years in prison after an emergency room doctor called the police when she sought help for what she said was a stillbirth but authorities said was a self-abortion. After serving more than three years in prison, her conviction was overturned.[47] (This happened while Vice President Mike Pence was governor of Indiana. Under his gubernatorial watch he reduced funding to Planned Parenthood, which resulted in the closure of non-abortion clinics that provided STD testing, contributing to a sharp rise in HIV infections in the state.)[48]

Author Scott Stern wrote about a shocking chapter in US history when the government devised a campaign (the "American plan") to eradicate sexually transmitted diseases by punishing the women believed to be at fault. Law enforcement officers literally grabbed women off the street who were considered dangers to the nation, including anyone deemed "promiscuous." When the women protested, some pointing out that they were virgins, authorities discounted their claims. Wrote Mr. Stern: "Indeed, for much of the twentieth century, tens, probably hundreds, of thousands of American women were detained and subjected to invasive examinations for sexually transmitted infections (the exams usually conducted by male physicians). These women were imprisoned in jails, 'detention houses,' or 'reformatories'—often without due process—and there treated with painful and ineffective remedies, such as injections of mercury."[49]

A year after candidate Trump's declaration about the need to punish women, a photo came out that seemed to reinforce the administration's attitude toward women's health. Tweeted by Vice President Pence, the picture showed President Trump and a group of male politicians sitting around a table, making decisions on women's healthcare policy, including discussions of how to reduce coverage for pregnancy and newborn care.[50]

A 2018 *New York Times* editorial observed that many women have felt unease over the future of their healthcare since the election of Donald Trump, "whose retrograde views on gender are straight out of the 1950s—or maybe the 1590s. . . . In policy terms, the administration has proved hostile to women on matters of reproductive health, not only chipping away at abortion rights but also curtailing access to birth control and peddling abstinence-only sex education. It also has worked to weaken protections for victims of sexual violence. At the same time, Republicans in Congress have been fighting to take away women's access to health care in general, targeting both Planned Parenthood and the Affordable Care Act."[51]

Breast cancer survivor Sascha Cohen—who was only thirty-three when she had a double mastectomy—wrote about the horror she felt when she read both her pathology report and her hospital bill. Her medical prognosis was grim, requiring months of treatment for an aggressive malignancy. Her medical expenses eventually topped half a million dollars, but, thanks to the Affordable Care Act, not only did her insurance cover everything, but if her cancer returns, "I won't have to choose between dying or going bankrupt. These protections and benefits are now at risk under a presidential administration hellbent on repealing the Affordable Care Act or weakening it through one policy change after another until it collapses. Thousands of women and men undergoing treatment for breast cancer (and millions more who have it on record as a preexisting condition) are vulnerable."[52]

Fomented in this political climate, certain fringe men's rights groups pose threats to women's safety by promoting furious antifeminist rhetoric; these groups blame women for men's social, health, and economic problems, sometimes encouraging violence against women. Op-ed columnist Gail Collins described a disturbing "political ethos that thinks grabbing private parts is fun and complaining about sexual assault is a threat to young manhood."[53]

The Centers for Disease Control and Prevention (CDC) reported that 36 percent of American women have experienced some form of sexual assault and that these survivors were more likely to later have heart disease and heart attacks.[54] A study published in the *Journal of the American Medical Association* (*JAMA*) in 2018 found that victims of sexual assault face long-term health problems beyond the injuries of the attack. The researchers concluded that sexual assault was associated with higher blood pressure, worsening mental health, and poorer sleep in midlife: "Efforts to improve women's health should target sexual harassment and assault prevention."[55]

A different kind of harassment has male-rights sects promoting false medical theories as part of their antifemale ideology. As pointed out in an article on growing concern over declines in sperm rates, certain groups are promulgating the idea that feminists are to blame. (Some experts believe the true culprits are environmental toxins like pesticides and possibly lifestyle hazards, such as smoking and obesity.) When reporter Nellie Bowles reached out to one online men's rights community, the head of the site responded on Twitter: "Tell your editor to stop being an idiot and reassign the article to a man. Then get in touch with me."[56]

These groups want to deny the voices of the #MeToo movement and to rewrite history to show that white men—rather than women—are the real forgotten victims. At the same time, the right seems to applaud men's anger while wanting women to remain quiet. But throughout society—including in medical settings—it is often women who are not seen, heard, or believed. Rebecca Traister, author of *Good and Mad: The Revolutionary Power of Women's Anger*, wrote in an essay that women are taught early in life "that if we express anger, we will not be taken seriously. We will sound 'childlike,' 'emotional,' 'unhinged,' 'hysterical.'"[57]

It's not uncommon for women with health problems to worry about being viewed as unstable or emotional. When television celebrity Maria Menounos sought help for neurological symptoms—which turned out to be a nonmalignant brain tumor—she was thankful to be quickly diagnosed and treated. No doubt aware of women whose physical symptoms were dismissed as psychological, she thanked her doctor on Twitter for "not making me feel like I was crazy."[58] Most of the women I spoke with felt such gratitude when they were diagnosed, even as they learned their condition was serious. Finally, someone paid attention.

This book focuses on areas of medicine where women are more likely to encounter problems in getting diagnosed and treated: neurology, cardiology, and chronic diseases. I also look at troubling patterns in gynecology, where patients have been particularly vulnerable. In addition, I examine the challenges that have faced female physicians striving to break into male-dominated medical specialties.

Dr. Miller of the Society for Women's Health Research told me that even with advances that have been made, there remains a "seeming disinterest in developing new therapeutics or new procedures or new medical devices or new diagnostic tests for women's health. . . . I think we have a lot of catching up to do."

She speculated that the problem is systemic, growing since the days when "women were actively discouraged from attending medical school, going into the sciences, looking into a microscope, and speaking up in math class."

To be clear, the point of this book is not about bashing healthcare providers of any gender. Some of my family members and dear friends are doctors, nurses, midwives, and public health advocates, and it's clear they want only the best for patients. Although I've had some bad experiences in medical settings, I've also had caring doctors and nurses heal me. And my husband and I will never forget—or be able to properly thank—the incredible medical team who saved our son's life.[59]

Simply put, I wanted to write this book because I was troubled and curious: Why, with all the technological advances now available, is it sometimes still challenging for a woman to get appropriate medical care? Why are women so frequently second-guessed when they offer evidence of a serious ailment? Why does it keep happening, and what can we do about it?

Dr. Paula Johnson framed the issue this way: "Why leave women's health to chance? This is a question that haunts those of us in science and medicine who believe that we are on the verge of being able to dramatically improve the health of women. . . . We know that women are not getting the full benefit of modern science and medicine today. We have the tools but we lack the collective will and momentum. Women's health is an equal rights issue as important as equal pay and it's an issue of the quality and the integrity of science and medicine."[60]

The #MeToo movement has proven how frequently women have been mistreated in every part of society and the workforce. The one place most of us have considered a safe haven is a medical facility—after all, doctors take an oath to do their best to help their patients and to not hurt them in the process. But harm can be a shape-shifter, inflicting damage even when none is intended. As the women in this book testify, when symptoms are dismissed, it can indeed cause lasting harm. It turns out healing is not possible unless doctors have the ability to listen and believe—without letting bias influence how they diagnose and treat the patients in their care.

I

ALL IN MY HEAD

I couldn't slide my right foot into a flip-flop.

It was June 2005 and I was rushing around, helping my daughter get ready for the senior prom. I thought that I had slipped my feet into the flip-flops by the front door as I hurried to my car in the driveway, but something felt wrong. I looked down and saw that my right foot was bare—the strap on the sandal must have snapped. But when I went back to retrieve the errant shoe, that wasn't the case. It seemed that the problem was not with the flip-flop, but with my suddenly funky foot.

I didn't make too much of this. I had been having weird neurological symptoms for nearly four years, mostly tingling and numbness in my arms and legs. When these symptoms first started, my primary care doctor diagnosed Guillain-Barré syndrome, an autoimmune disease that attacks the nervous system. He referred me to a neurologist at West Hills Hospital in the San Fernando Valley. That doctor examined me and said I had a Guillain-Barré-*like* virus and that I would recover in a few weeks.

When that didn't happen, I went for another opinion with a neurologist at UCLA. He agreed with the original diagnosis.

"Should I have some kind of tests?" I timidly asked.

The doctor chuckled and said something along the lines of: "I could order all kinds of tests and have you spend lots of money, but it's not necessary."

I didn't protest. After all, *he* was the highly regarded physician, and I grew up in an environment when patients, especially women, would never question a medical professional. Plus, I've always hated going to the doctor and any kind of medical procedure. (Seriously, I get nervous at the dentist during a routine cleaning.) So if two neurologists were telling me that I would recuperate without intervention, I was more than happy to believe them. Besides, life was busy, with two teenagers, a husband who had a high-stress job, in-laws and extended family who visited several times a year, and a writing career that demanded many hours.

And eventually, I honestly couldn't tell if I was better or if not feeling right had become my new normal. At one point I wondered if what I was experiencing might be menopause. I called my mother-in-law to ask: "Do hot flashes feel like tingling in your limbs?"

"No," she explained. "You actually get hot during a hot flash."

So I carried on, a somewhat altered version of myself, until the day I ended up minus a shoe. My husband, Stu, urged me to check back in with the UCLA neurologist. As it happened, I recently had had an inconclusive mammogram and ultrasound and had scheduled a follow-up appointment at the UCLA Breast Center. Stu took the day off of work to accompany me. As long as we were going to be on campus, I took his advice and made an appointment with the neurologist to discuss this new symptom.

After I described my flip-flop malfunction, the doctor had me sit on his exam table and close my eyes. Then he manipulated the toes on my right foot and asked whether the digits were up or down. I had no clue.

"Have you ever had an MRI?" the doctor asked.

Within the hour, I was taking my first ride in an enclosed metal tube. The MRI technician asked what kind of music I wanted to listen to—a pointless question, I soon learned, because the exam was so noisy it was impossible to hear anything but the clamor of the machine.

When the test was over, we met a friend for lunch, which left me feeling queasy. (Most likely the nausea came from the contrast dye used in the imaging. But I was then an MRI virgin and didn't know that reaction was possible.) After lunch I headed to the Breast Center for my appointment. A physician's assistant went over the mammogram and ultrasound and assured me that everything was fine—proving my theory that the thing you're worried about usually is not the thing that you *should* be worried about.

Suddenly my pager began to blow up. (This was before we all had cell phones.) I looked at the number and saw it was the neurologist. He wanted me to return to the imaging center pronto for an additional scan.

Then I should bring the discs back to his office. It was already late in the day, but he would wait.

We high-tailed it back to the imaging center (and by *high-tail* I mean we slogged through Wilshire Boulevard rush-hour traffic). As soon as I checked in, they hurried me to the exam room, where I again was placed in the MRI machine. This time no one asked what kind of music I favored.

About halfway through the exam, the technician came into the room. "So, um," she said. "Do you get a lot of headaches?"

"No, I never get headaches," I answered. "Why, what do you see?"

She backed up toward the door: "Oh, um, why don't we let the professionals answer that."

She bolted, and the clanging and banging of the MRI machine resumed. Two thoughts crossed my mind. One: Technician, work on your subtlety skills. Two: I am so screwed.

Back in the neurologist's office, we sat silently by his computer as he inserted the discs and waited for the information to download. Images of my brain appeared, and there, at the top, was a large, white circle. I was a terrible science student, but even I knew that blob probably wasn't supposed to be there.

The doctor clicked on different views and said I most likely had a benign meningioma (a tumor that forms on the membranes covering the brain and spinal cord), a word I had never heard before, which would require surgery. He added that there were going to be some challenges. For starters, the tumor was very big, roughly the size of a baseball. And it had become entangled with a major artery supplying blood to the brain.

"You want to get someone good to do this," he said.

I no doubt was experiencing psychic shock. What I remember most clearly was how surprised and relieved I was to hear the word *benign*. I had always assumed brain tumor meant cancer. I also was stunned at how large the thing in my head was. I wondered—how long had this tumor been growing undetected?

Before we left, the neurologist walked me over to his assistant and asked her to arrange appointments with two renowned Los Angeles neurosurgeons: one at UCLA and a second, Dr. Keith Black, at Cedars-Sinai Medical Center. The assistant made a joke about wanting to deliver my chart to Dr. Black in person. I was too dazed by the events of the day to process what she was saying. The neurologist explained that Dr. Black is considered to be very handsome.

At least there was that to look forward to.

* * *

Two days later we were back at UCLA to meet with the first recommended neurosurgeon. The appointment was scheduled for 2:30 p.m., but we sat in the waiting room until close to 4:00 p.m. When my name finally was called, we headed to his exam room. As we approached the door, it opened, and a woman came out, accompanied by a man and a young boy. She was sobbing inconsolably.

We entered the room. The doctor was sitting in front of the scans of my brain, which were displayed on a light box. My husband and I sat down, facing him. He leaned back in his chair and looked at us with what I can only describe as a sneer. There was a long, awkward silence.

Finally, staring at the ceiling, he spoke, sounding incredibly bored, as if this was all a nuisance: "What do you want me to tell you?"

It was a startling question, asked in such a rude way that I'm pretty sure my jaw dropped open. Stu calmly responded, "We'd like you to evaluate Emily's MRI and hear what treatment you would recommend."

The doctor looked at the MRI and turned his attention to me.

"We're going to cut your head open like a pumpkin, take off the top, put it over here, take out the tumor, and put the top back on."

As he spoke, his hands mimed the activity of carving open a pumpkin and removing the top.

My older sister, who is a nurse/midwife, had warned me that some neurosurgeons have strange personalities. But this was more than bad bedside manner—here was a doctor in a position of power being deliberately cruel to a vulnerable patient. (Looking back, I'm certain he would not have addressed a male patient in such a cavalier manner.) My husband pressed the neurosurgeon for specifics, while I sat silent and stunned. At one point, the doctor commented on how many questions my husband was asking.

"Occupational hazard," my husband replied.

"What do you mean?" the neurosurgeon asked.

Stu explained that he was a reporter for the *Los Angeles Times*. This got the doctor's attention. There was an immediate shift in his demeanor.

He bragged to my husband that he recently had had dinner with a top suit from the paper. And he stopped comparing my head to a squash.

Then he began to discuss my surgical options in a serious and respectful manner. In his view, I would need two operations. The first would be to deal with the artery that was tangled up in the tumor, to prevent a major hemorrhage. The day after that procedure, a craniotomy would be performed to remove the tumor.

He wanted us to sign up on the spot, but my husband said we were planning to get a second opinion from another neurosurgeon. The doctor guessed that we were headed to Cedars-Sinai—without naming names, he began to bash the surgeons there. It was shocking—as well as inappropriate and unprofessional.

My head was spinning, and I was feeling scared, desperate, and hopeless. I couldn't wait to get out of there.

A few days later we went to Cedars-Sinai. As we entered the waiting room, Stu suddenly said, "Hey, Oprah!" He pointed to a large plaque on the wall, listing donors to the Maxine Dunitz Neurosurgical Institute. One of the names was Oprah Winfrey. I have always admired her. Seeing her name on the plaque gave me a lift. I figured this was a good omen.

I checked in and was informed I would need to pay a facility fee, which would not be covered by insurance. This was my first encounter with such a charge. Being already dazed, I didn't quite get what the fee was for, but I paid up, then went to the restroom—where there was no toilet paper. Clearly, the facility fee didn't cover the facilities.[1]

A few minutes after I returned to the waiting area, a physician's assistant escorted us to an exam room. She explained that Dr. Black was reviewing my scans and would be in shortly. When Dr. Black came in, I liked him right away. He had a pleasant manner and was able to translate the complex medical situation into terms I could grasp. He explained that the tumor was too big for radiation treatment and that surgery was the only option. (This was the first time I understood that if the tumor had been detected at an earlier stage, surgery might have been avoided in favor of radiation. Again I wondered—how long had this mass been growing undiagnosed?)

I asked Dr. Black about the two-part surgery that the UCLA doctor had recommended. Dr. Black emphatically said, "No." In his opinion, this would put me at risk for a stroke. He said the problematic artery would be dealt with during the craniotomy.

Minutes into the consult with Dr. Black I knew that I wanted him to do the surgery. In addition to his stellar reputation, he had just the right combination of confidence and compassion. Most of all, he made me feel hopeful that I could get through this health crisis in one piece and eventually would be able to return to my normal life.

I asked Dr. Black how long I would be out of commission after the surgery. He said it would take about a month to recover. Also, because the tumor was on the motor strip for my right foot, I would need physical therapy to relearn how to walk.

Calendars were consulted and I was told I could have the operation either the very next week, or in six weeks. Usually, I would want to get something I'm dreading over with as soon as possible. But this time I chose to delay. My rationale for doing this can be explained in four words: Bed Bath & Beyond.

Our daughter, Amy, was leaving soon to start her freshman year of college, and I had been looking forward to doing the dorm shop-a-thon with her. We had amassed a huge pile of coupons with which to fill a shopping cart with all the necessities. If I had the surgery right away, I wouldn't be able to help her get ready for school. So the surgery was scheduled for six weeks out.

In addition to helping my daughter prepare for college, one of my daily activities during this presurgery time was a little game I thought of as: "Let's Call the Insurance Company and Ask How Much I'm Going to Pay."

Here's how it worked: Every day I would ask a customer service representative if he or she could please give me an estimate on how much my copay for the surgery would be. After all, anyone who's ever been in a hospital knows that it costs roughly $100 every time you pee. So I was curious.

Each time I called I got a new version of my benefits. One of my favorite conversations went like this:

Customer Service Rep: You need to make sure that everyone who touches you in the hospital is part of your plan.

Me: I'm going to be unconscious for more than five hours. How's that going to work?

Customer Service Rep: It is still your responsibility.

I knew I was fortunate to have good health insurance, thanks to my husband's job. I also knew that I would never again be able to purchase health insurance, because I now had a monster of a preexisting condition. (This fact led Stu to leave a job he loved in 2008, when the *Los Angeles Times* was on shaky financial ground and offering buyouts. He decided to take what was rumored to be the last buyout that would allow employees to keep paying for the company insurance plan. This was before the Affordable Care Act, which gave people like me the right to buy health insurance.)

I never did get an accurate estimate of the surgery cost and eventually I stopped caring. My head was in a weird place, no pun intended. It reminded me of postpartum depression, except this was precraniotomy depression. The hardest part was announcing my bad health news. I started to dread the ringing of the phone.

"I hear you have a tumor!" began one call from a well-meaning relative.

It was difficult for me to tell even my closest friends. And I certainly did not want to tell people I was working for, especially in the entertainment industry. Over the years, in addition to being a freelance journalist, I've written and sold a few scripts. For the most part, this has been fun, as well as a way to help both our kids graduate from college debt-free. In the months prior to my surgery I was working on a script with a small production company. I meant to tell the producers that I was about to have my head sawed open, but I just couldn't think of how to work it into the conversation. Plus, everyone knows you can't be old or sick in Hollywood, especially if you're a woman—and now I was all three. (In hindsight, I probably could have just let slip that I was having "work done" at Cedars-Sinai and no one would have blinked.)

As the surgery date approached, I focused on getting the house in order and cooking food for the freezer, sort of like the nesting you do before having a baby. I've saved all my desk diaries through the years. That month I composed a detailed to-do list containing twelve items, four having to do with laundry, including "ironing." Ironing? Really?

At night, the gravity of what I was facing would hit me. Our son, Josh, a recent college graduate, had moved back home to help out. He is the funniest guy I know and always makes me laugh, no matter what is going on. Every evening after dinner, Josh (who now is a television comedy writer and producer) would take a look at my face and comment, "Time for Mom's meltdown."

A week before the surgery I went for a physical at Cedars-Sinai. The nice internist doing the exam asked if I drank alcohol. "Not really," I answered. His joking reply: "Maybe you should."

During the appointment a compassionate nurse gently explained what would happen before, during, and after the operation. She gave me a giant three-ring binder titled *Information for Patients Undergoing a Biopsy or Craniotomy for a Brain Tumor*. Every time I opened the binder, I started to panic. (In fact, it is only recently that I've been able read it all the way through.)

Coincidentally, the wife of one of my husband's friends and colleagues at the newspaper had recently had meningioma surgery at Cedars-Sinai with Dr. Black's team. Her husband sent word to Stu that I could call her, which I did. Her surgery had gone very well (in fact, she traveled to Europe a month after the operation, which was great to hear.) She gave me some good practical advice, such as: if I colored my hair (yes), get it done before the surgery, because I wouldn't be able to do it for a while after. And she also offered this comforting overview: I was going to be treated by some of the best neurosurgeons in the country, and they were going to take great care of me.

When we hung up the phone, I looked at the clock and was mortified to see that I had kept her on the line for nearly an hour. To this day I still remember and appreciate her kindness and patience with my many questions.

The day before the surgery I went to Cedars-Sinai for a specialized preop MRI, intended to give the doctors a detailed road map of inside my head. Little circular markers (called *fiducials*) that resembled Life Savers candies were affixed all over my face; I had to keep them in place and not get them wet.

When we got back home late that afternoon, we discovered that the air conditioner had decided that this was a good day to stop working. Outside, it was over 100 degrees (normal for August in the San Fernando Valley), and inside it was even hotter. I hoped sweaty fiducials were not going to present a problem. All I could think of was that I would be recovering from brain surgery in a steaming house. I called a repairman we had used once before and begged him to come out the next day. I explained that I would be having surgery, but we would leave a door open for him. (He did come out and fix the air conditioner, and he never charged us a penny. I'm including this information in case you believe there are no decent people left on earth.)

I didn't even bother trying to sleep that night. I emptied the dishwasher and then gave myself a pedicure. I wrote a letter to my husband and kids, as well as a medical directive giving the doctors permission to donate my "good parts" if things didn't go well.

Early the next morning, we drove to the hospital.

* * *

The neurosurgical waiting room was bustling with patients and their families. When patients' names were called, volunteers escorted them out. A white-haired, grandmotherly woman with a thick accent came to get me. She waited while I hugged my family, then she took me by the hand. For an elderly woman, she had a surprisingly strong grip. I wondered if perhaps someone had once tried to run away at this juncture. There was a door beckoning with an "Exit" sign. I could see out the large picture windows to the street below, where pedestrians were starting their days. I desperately wanted to join them, especially the people heading for coffee.

I was delivered to a preop area. A nurse gave me a gown and a bed. An anesthesiologist appeared. He examined my arms and scowled, clearly annoyed that my veins were not cooperating. (*Give me a break*, I thought. *I haven't had anything to eat or drink since midnight.*) Eventually, he found a vein that worked and he hooked me up to an IV. As I was wheeled off to the operating room, the magic potion kicked in, and I felt fuzzy and relaxed.

The operating room was abuzz with bright lights and lots of activity. I recognized Dr. Black and was happy to see him.

"Hey, Dr. Black!" I exclaimed in a cheerful, goofy way.

He gave my shoulder a firm, friendly squeeze. I appreciated that gesture—something about it was so reassuring.

This was my first surgery. I had heard that when you wake up it seems as if no time has passed. That was the sense I had when I suddenly became aware of a voice calling my name. As I came to, Dr. Black was there, saying, "You're cured."

I must have quickly gone back to sleep. When I opened my eyes again I was in a recovery room with other patients. Nearby a man was groaning, in terrible pain, from back surgery. Across the way, doctors and nurses were working on a woman, another brain tumor patient, who appeared to be in serious trouble. "We need to intubate," I heard someone say. There was a flurry of activity until she was stabilized.

I dozed off, and when I woke up my family was there. I was surprised to learn it was late afternoon. I asked them what they had eaten for lunch. They told me about the friends who had sat with them in the waiting room.

I was feeling great! As I was wheeled to my room, I threw up all over everything. The nurses assured me this was normal, most likely a reaction to the motion, the anesthesia, the pain meds, or the fact that the inside of my head had been rearranged.

A cot was provided so my husband could stay with me. I was cleaned up and squeezy things were wrapped around my legs to prevent blood clots. (The real name is *intermittent pneumatic compression devices*— basically, they are leg coverings that inflate and deflate with an air pump.)

I was given steroids to reduce brain swelling, as well as a choice of pain meds. I've always been sensitive to medications and worried that anything heavy-duty would make me vomit again, so I opted for Tylenol.

Surprisingly, there wasn't a lot of head pain—mostly pressure. The Tylenol didn't really relieve this, but I stuck with it anyway. Because too much acetaminophen can cause liver failure, the nurses were very careful with the dosage.

I can't say enough about how wonderful the neurosurgical nurses were. While a surgeon can save your life in the operating room, it's the nurses who keep you alive once you are wheeled out. Not only did they take great care of me, but they also came to the aid of my husband— during the night he developed an itchy rash from the high-octane detergent used to wash the sheets. Whenever the nurses came in to check on me, they examined him, too, giving him different ointments to relieve his itching.

I only was scheduled to spend two nights in the hospital. During the second night, I was hungry and was offered Jell-O. As soon as I finished the small cup, I began to feel weird shaking throughout my body. This intensified until every muscle, from head to toe, was having uncontrollable, violent spasms.

Naturally, this occurred at 2:00 a.m., when the doctors patrolling the floor were new-arrival residents. A posse of them stood by the bed and watched me shiver and shake. They clearly did not want to wake the attending physician, who must have threatened them with physical harm if they interrupted his nap. After observing me for a while, the leader of the pack intoned, "We don't know what's wrong with you, but we think the problem is all in your head."

He wasn't trying to be funny.

My nurse speculated that the steroids were causing the muscle spasms. I actually thought it was the combination of the sugar from the Jell-O and the steroids. Eventually the shaking stopped. The next day, when I had one spoonful of pudding with lunch, I immediately felt small muscle flutters again in my stomach. I stopped eating sweets while on the steroids, although no one else bought my sugar-steroid hypothesis.

Because of this episode, I had a chest X-ray and an MRI, both normal, and was kept in the hospital for an additional day. I was examined several times by Dr. Black and other members of his team, who cleared me to go home three days after surgery.

I was sent packing with a cane to help me walk. At first, even that aid wasn't enough. Stu had to practically carry me from the car into the house. It was great to be home, but I had three immediate concerns: food, coffee, and hairy legs.

The first problem was solved by our loyal and amazing friends, who brought over delicious meals to get us through the first few days. Morning coffee was another hurdle. I've always been an early riser, and a latte is how I start the day. I'm a fussbudget in the kitchen, starting with that first cup of coffee, which I like with a cloud of foamed milk on top. My husband had been by my side through this whole ordeal, and I didn't want to burden him now with having to learn how to make my coffee. Also, the guy can't cook. His mother, may she rest in peace, had amazing culinary talents, but she never shared those skills with her two sons. I've known my husband for more than forty years, and in all that time, he's cooked dinner once. It was while we were dating, when he threw some brown rice and veggies into a pot. We affectionately refer to this as his seduction dinner.

If I wanted my morning latte, I was on my own. One hurdle was getting downstairs. By grasping the wall and bannister, and by going very slowly, I could make it to the first floor, where I collapsed onto the living room sofa. After I recovered from that trek, I used the cane to go into the dining room, where I turned a chair into a walker to get into the kitchen. There, I was able to make coffee and foam the milk. When I got tired, I could plunk myself down in the chair. Problem solved.

Hairy legs were another issue. One of the directives in the recovery packet was not to lower my head for a month. It's hard to shave your legs if you can't put your head down to see what you're doing. I asked our daughter, Amy, to help me out for a few weeks, until she left for college. I figured she owed me—for the first three years of her life she had been permanently attached to my legs. When she was a toddler, if I left her for three minutes to go into the bathroom, she would collapse in a puddle of tears. (She grew up to be the most independent young woman I know. She's now a fearless investigative journalist.) When I asked her to assist with my hirsute limbs, she thought it over and responded, "Okay, but only below the knees." Fair enough.

A week after the surgery, I had an appointment at Dr. Black's office to have the stitches removed. I still was unsteady on my feet, so we arranged for a wheelchair. In the procedure room, a physician's assistant had me move to a regular chair rather than having me lie down. This was an educational moment for both of us. The lesson we learned: It's probably not a great idea for someone fresh out of brain surgery to sit upright for an extended period of time while stitches are removed.

A few minutes into the procedure, the room started to spin.

"I think I'm going to pass out," I calmly announced, which I then proceeded to do.

When I came to, I was face-to-face with a very handsome EMT. (Question: Why is every male and female firefighter and EMT in Los Angeles so good-looking?) He wanted to know if I had peed myself. I did a quick inspection and determined that I had not. (If I had, that could have been indication of a seizure.)

I was carried off, put in an ambulance, and driven around the block to the busy Cedars-Sinai emergency room. Once I was settled in a cubicle there, a friendly nurse took down all of my information. When he heard that I had had surgery the prior week with Dr. Black, he said: "Dr. Black is amazing. He can remove half your brain and you'll still be fine."

An ER doctor checked me out and said that I had fainted, most likely due to something called the *vasovagal reflex*. This was my first experience with fainting. I learned that the large vagal nerve descends from the spinal cord and has nerve endings throughout the body, including the neck, chest, and abdomen. It is part of the autonomic nervous system, which regulates heart rate and blood pressure.

"The vasovagal reflex is mediated by this nerve. In certain sensitive individuals, exposure to shocking stimuli (pain, emotional distress, anxiety, and fear) results in activation of the vagal nerve's action, which then causes a reduction in heart rate and blood pressure," Dr. Sam S. Torbati, an emergency medicine specialist at Cedars-Sinai, told me for an article I later wrote about fainting. [2]

I also could have passed out simply because I was sitting upright, which allowed the blood to flow downward. It was a warm day and I was dehydrated and exhausted—all of these may have been contributing factors.

As soon as I was lying down, with my feet up, I felt fine. By the time Dr. Black arrived in the emergency room, my primary symptom was embarrassment for causing such a to-do. I also felt guilty that he had been dragged away from his important work. He examined me and agreed that I had fainted and that nothing more serious was going on. He asked what I wanted to do.

"I really just want to go home, have something to eat, and go to bed," I answered.

Every doctor, nurse, aide, and technician within earshot echoed this sentiment, with affirmations like: "Sounds like a plan . . . Amen to that . . . Yes!"

* * *

Although I was expecting to feel back to normal within a month, that wasn't the case. Despite physical therapy, my right foot remained mostly numb. I eventually relearned to walk, but my foot always felt weird. It seemed to be a kind of neuropathy, similar to what some people with diabetes experience. Physical therapy didn't help. I later learned the permanent numbness probably was caused by scar tissue on the brain's motor nerve for my foot.

I didn't feel comfortable driving because I couldn't tell, without looking, if my foot was on the gas or brake pedal. So I decided to enroll in an adaptive driving program offered at Northridge Hospital in the San Fernando Valley.

I was sent information about the program and learned that on the first day I would be given a written test to evaluate my driving readiness. I've always been a terrible test taker (and I have the low SAT scores to prove it), so I was nervous the morning of the exam. I drank two strong cups of coffee, hoping to be extra alert. Instead, I was jumpy and ended up with a bad stomachache. It was a cool morning, and I wore a heavy sweater. But in the exam room, the heat was blasting, and I was so uncomfortable that I had trouble concentrating.

If this sounds like I am making excuses for my poor showing on the test—that's exactly what I'm doing. The director of the program frowned as she graded my paper.

"What kind of cognitive impairment did they say you have?" she asked midway through.

"None," I said. "My right foot is kind of numb. I can't feel the car pedals."

She looked at me as if I were delusional. "Well," she said. "Once they start messing with your gray matter . . ."

The bad news was that the test suggested I had suffered cognitive impairment. But the good news was that I was okay to drive in Los Angeles, where the bar apparently is low.

In fairness to the program director, I actually think she may have picked up on something I wasn't aware of at the time. In the first months after surgery I would get overwhelmed by too much information hitting me all at once. Even a long phone call was disorienting. An occupational therapist I saw compared it to a computer crashing. She called it "brain overload," an accurate description. For example, when I went into a grocery store, the music, bright lights, and people moving around were more than I could handle and triggered a kind of panic attack (a disorder I never had before the surgery). Over time this went away, but I think the craniotomy did leave me with a bit of a processing problem. Sometimes, I'll think one word and say something else. The other day, I was ordering jeans over the phone. When the salesperson asked what credit card I wanted to use, I said Mastercard and gave her the number. But I was holding a Visa card.

At the driving program, once I was cleared for takeoff, I scheduled classes with an instructor, a pleasant middle-aged man with nerves of steel. I nearly killed both of us multiple times when I was trying out cars operated with hand controls. I just could not get the hang of those devices. There was one other option, which the program discouraged: driving with your left foot. In this scenario, the gas and brake pedals are flipped. Your right foot rests on a little platform and your left foot does all the work. Apparently, a lot of people get confused in stressful driving situations and hit the gas when they mean to slam on the brakes. But I didn't appear to have that problem, maybe because I had grown dependent on my left foot, and using it to drive felt natural.

There was a company in Canoga Park that could install the adaptive equipment in my old Volvo. They've since left the area. My car now is an antique, but I refuse to give it up since there's no one nearby who can adapt a new car for me. I'm sure our neighbors hate my ancient auto, which lowers property values every time it's parked on the street. Even with the adaptive equipment, I don't feel all that comfortable on the road and stick to what I call "bubble driving"—the neighborhood grocery store, the local library, or my son and daughter-in-law's nearby house. If I have an appointment "over the hill," Stu always rearranges his schedule to take me.

* * *

After the surgery I went back to the UCLA neurologist for periodic checkups. At first I had to have an MRI every three months, then every six months, then annually. Finally, I graduated to every two years. Each time, the neurologist sent me an e-mail with the welcome results, based on a radiologist's report: "No evidence of tumor recurrence."

I had all of my imaging tests done at Cedars-Sinai. I liked the technicians there, and the scans could be done early on Sunday mornings, a nice convenience. During the procedure, I would try to think about something fun to do afterward. (Top of the list: cinnamon rolls and coffee at Sweet Lady Jane, a West Hollywood bakery.)

There was camaraderie among the patients in the ladies' dressing room. After we put on our hospital gowns, we would sit in a waiting area until it was our turn. Sometimes we talked about why we were there, but mostly it was just friendly chitchat.

One time when I was in the dressing room changing, I heard a woman in the stall next to me start sobbing. I exited my stall and listened. The crying grew louder. I wasn't sure what to do—she hadn't seen me and thought she was alone. Finally, when the crying grew worse, I asked if I could call someone for her. She stopped crying and, in a calm voice, said she was fine, thank you. I was seated in the waiting area when she came out of the dressing room. She was young and fashionable, with skinny red jeans and a cute blond bob (which, looking back, probably was a wig). If you passed her on the street, you would never know she had just been crying in an MRI dressing room.

* * *

We had been hearing good things about the local branch of the large HMO, Kaiser Permanente, and in 2014 we decided to change insurance plans. One of my first appointments was with a neurologist. My goal for the appointment was to convince him that I now could have an MRI every three years, instead of every two. I dreaded the exams. I'm not claustrophobic—which is a problem for some people having the scans—but I'm paranoid about the possible side effects of the contrast dye, so I liked the idea of spacing out the procedure as much as possible. (When I first started having MRIs, there was no pre-imaging lab work. Now you have to have a blood test to check kidney function, because researchers discovered that some patients with undetected kidney disease could have a catastrophic reaction to the contrast dye. One of my grandmothers and an aunt died of kidney disease, which makes me cautious of any potential threat to these organs. And Israeli researchers did a study that concluded the dye could be dangerous because it stays in your body for a long time—or possibly forever.)[3]

I met with a Kaiser Woodland Hills neurologist who ignored my suggestion to delay the next MRI; it had been two years since my last exam and he insisted I have one now. Grumpy, I scheduled the procedure. The day after the test, I had a meeting for a television project. Two producers were interested in developing a kids' TV show for a boy band and I had been hired to come up with a concept.

Because the meeting was far away, Stu drove me. He dropped me off at what I thought was the entrance, but when I checked in, the guard informed me that this was not the right gate. It was a nice day and I had arrived early, so I decided to walk to the correct gate.

As I made my way around a corner, I realized I had taken a wrong turn and was now lost. Just then my cell phone rang. I didn't recognize the number but thought it must be someone calling to say the meeting was delayed.

Instead, a woman's voice informed me that I needed to make an appointment right away at the Kaiser Sunset neurosurgery department to discuss the meningioma.

I stopped walking.

"Excuse me?"

She repeated the information. I told her I would call her back. I hung up and called my husband.

"I can't find the entrance. And the meningioma is back."

Stu told me not to move; he would find me. A few minutes later he appeared, and I got in the car. I wanted to call and cancel the meeting, but he convinced me to go through with it because people were waiting. We would deal with Kaiser after the meeting.

He drove me to the correct entrance. I checked in with a guard and was directed to the meeting room. To this day, I can't tell you who was there. Maybe there were three or four men and two women? Some of them had British accents. I still have no idea how most of these people were connected to the boy band.

I sat next to one of the producers who had hired me. There was friendly banter in the room, and we listened to the band's new single. Then I presented the concept pitch and somehow got through it. It was an out-of-body experience. On the way out, the producer I knew remarked, "You seemed really nervous."

I considered it a victory that I hadn't thrown up during the meeting.

Back in the car, I returned the Kaiser call and reached the nurse for the neurologist I had seen the week before. She was surprised to hear that the doctor had not informed me of the MRI results. In fact, he had left the office for the day, dumping the bad-news phone call on her. While the neurologist deserves kudos for insisting I go for the MRI, it goes without saying that he should have called me himself with the results.

The nurse apologized profusely, obviously upset with what the doctor had done. After making sure that I wasn't driving, she pulled up the MRI scan on her computer and examined the image. She told me the tumor was really small. That made me feel better, but I still couldn't believe this was happening again.

* * *

A few days later, Stu and I were in a waiting room for the Kaiser neuro-surgery department. When we checked in, a nurse explained that a group of specialists (called the Tumor Board) were reviewing my case and all of my scans.

After about forty-five minutes a serious, youngish neurosurgeon met with us. He showed me the most recent Kaiser MRI scan and pointed out the tumor.

"It's roughly the size of a pea," he said.

He explained that the doctors had gone over all of my past MRIs from Cedars-Sinai and had discovered that the tumor regrowth was actually visible on the scans taken as far back as 2009.

Wait, what? The tumor was there five years ago and no one had caught it?

The doctor showed me those prior scans where the beginnings of the new tumor could be seen. How on earth had this been missed? I was stunned.

If we had not switched insurance plans, would the tumor have continued to go undetected for years, so that eventually I would have had to have another craniotomy? I'll never know. What I do know is this: A hardworking radiologist at Kaiser Permanente Woodland Hills Medical Center spotted the tumor regrowth while it was pea-sized. Because he did his job so well, I could avoid having a craniotomy and instead have a one-day radiation treatment.

* * *

I met with three different Kaiser neurosurgeons who all said the same thing—the time for "watchful waiting" had passed. Left to its own devices, the meningioma was going to keep growing. So I scheduled the radiation appointment for the following week.

The treatment started early in the morning with a CT scan. Then a special plastic mask for me to wear during radiation was molded over my face. This needed several hours to set.

The radiation session wasn't until the afternoon. Stu and I took a walk around the neighborhood, then headed back to our car to get the picnic lunch I had packed. We had heard there was a rooftop lounge area, but it turned out this was designated for employees. However, a nurse said it was fine for us to hang out there, so we ate and enjoyed the view of the Hollywood sign. After lunch I stopped by the pharmacy to pick up the antiseizure medication I needed to take before the procedure and for a week after. (I've never had seizures, but with most brain procedures, this medication is prescribed.)

* * *

If you're ever feeling sorry for yourself, go hang out in the waiting room of a radiation oncology department.

At the Kaiser Sunset building, in the early afternoon on Wednesday, March 12, 2014, this department was packed with patients. Most of these people had cancer. The lucky ones were like me, there for one round of stereotactic radiosurgery.

I was confused by the system, which resembled the DMV, with numbers scrolling overhead near the ceiling. I asked a teenager seated nearby how the process worked, and he explained that when it was my turn, my number would appear and I would be called in.

He was a sweet boy, a high school senior. His world recently had imploded when he learned he had a malignant brain tumor. He showed me the outlines of the implanted shunt on the side of his head. He had difficulty talking but was still understandable. He already had been through surgery and chemotherapy; he especially hated the radiation sessions and couldn't wait to get home and play video games. Even though he didn't have a date, he was looking forward to the senior prom that spring. Right before his name was called, he took out his driver's license and showed me the photo. I think he wanted me to understand how handsome and popular he used to be, before the brain tumor destroyed his life.

Anyone battling brain cancer or caring for a loved one with the disease would be justified in telling me to stop complaining about my medical journey. A malignant brain tumor (more common in men than in women) is one of the most devastating diagnoses a person can get.

As I sat in the waiting room, I realized that many of the people who were there were friends because they had been having Wednesday afternoon appointments together for weeks or even months. As one woman came back into the waiting room after her session, she was greeted with applause and cheers at having come to the end of her radiation treatments.

When my number appeared on the scroll, one of the neurosurgeons from the Tumor Board came to get me. He asked how I was doing. I said I was tired, either from the antiseizure medication or because I hadn't slept much the night before.

The doctor looked at me for a beat, clearly puzzled. "Oh . . . did you have butterflies?" he asked.

I like this doctor a lot. He's a kind man and it seems he's very good at what he does. So I'm going to blame his medical school education: Clearly, some neurosurgeons are not taught that while zapping someone's brain is just another day at the office for them, it's traumatic for patients.

Butterflies? More like freaking out.

I was taken to the treatment room and put on a narrow gurney. The plastic mask that had been made in the morning was clamped onto my face. The doctor said the procedure would take about thirty minutes, and he left the room.

What transpired was like something out of a sci-fi movie. The gurney was raised and lowered and spun around as beams crisscrossed the room. It seemed like a lot of *lights, camera, action!* to neutralize a teeny tumor. While all this was going on, I did simple subtraction. It's a little exercise I do from time to time to make sure my brain is still working. (Start at 100, then subtract by 7, trying to do it quickly, all the way down to zero. Or start at 112, then subtract by 9. Not sure my father—the late Meyer Dwass, who was a brilliant math professor—would have been impressed by this, but I'm always happy when I can do it.)

When the room finally stopped spinning, the mask was removed and I went to the nursing station. There I was given a dose of steroids to reduce the possibility of brain swelling. Other than being wiped out, I didn't feel any different. My only complaint was that my left eye seemed to have been scratched by the mask. The nurse gave me some eye drops to take home, along with a list of precautions and possible side effects of the procedure.

Under the heading "Why Radiosurgery Works" was the revelation that "the mechanisms in reducing tumor size following radiosurgery is not entirely clear."

Okay.

The goal of the treatment is not to make the tumor disappear, but to weaken its mojo "at the molecular level. While it does not remove the lesion, radiosurgery inactivates the cells so they are unable to divide."

There is a lot that can go wrong after brain radiation. There can be swelling, requiring more steroids; the beams can cause brain tissue to die (necrosis), which then must be removed surgically; the radiation can cause new tumors to grow.

A month after the treatment, I had a follow-up appointment at which a young doctor I had never met before examined me. I told her I was feeling fine, which didn't seem to impress her. She explained that the possible bad effects of radiosurgery still could happen—I would be vulnerable for swelling and necrosis for at least a year. And all bets were off on whether or not the radiation might one day cause other tumors to grow.

Fortunately—so far, anyway—I haven't experienced any of those issues. After my radiation treatment, I was back to having MRIs every three months, then six months, then annually. After my last exam, I graduated to every two years. Unlike the old days, when I would await word from the neurologist by e-mail, I now have a different system in place: The morning of the exam, Stu drives me to Kaiser Sunset, about forty-five minutes away in good traffic. After the scan, the results are immediately uploaded. I then head over to meet with one of the neurosurgeons who was part of the radiation team. Over the years, he's become one of my favorite doctors.

I appreciate that, as this doctor walks into the room, he greets me with a smile and says, "Everything looks good."

Then he goes to the computer and pulls up the scan. Together, we look at my brain.

2

ALL IN HER HEAD

When I met Byrdie Lifson-Pompan, the first thing that struck me was how much she resembles the actress Sandra Bullock. Only after talking with her for a while did I realize that the left side of her beautiful face does not move.

Her problems started in 2003, when she was thirty-seven and one of the busiest executives in Hollywood. It's an understatement to say she had a lot on her plate. She was a top literary agent and partner at Creative Artists Agency, where she represented superstar clients like writer/directors Richard LaGravenese and Paul Haggis. In addition to her intense and constant career demands, she was a caring mom for two young children and a devoted daughter to elderly parents. Her father had just been diagnosed with a rare form of prostate cancer and given six weeks to live. She was a woman used to getting things done and was determined to find a doctor who could treat him. Her own health was pretty far down her list of daily concerns. When she experienced a small facial spasm, she didn't make too much of it.

"You know that little twitch that happens under your eye? You can feel it, and you keep saying to people, can you see this? And they say, 'No, I don't see anything.' You can feel that flutter and it's super annoying," she recalled when we talked in the living room of her lovely Los Angeles home.

She tried to ignore it, but then "the twitch started to get a little worse and I started to have some headaches. Then I developed a noticeable paralysis starting in the left side of my face. I went to my internist. He sent me to a neurologist. Given that I was so busy at work and I had these really demanding clients . . . and my children were young and my father had just been diagnosed—the neurologist chalked it up to stress and prescribed Xanax."

The antianxiety drug didn't help with the facial spasms—although Byrdie joked that she nevertheless enjoyed the false sense of calm it gave her. When the strange symptoms didn't abate, she went back to the doctor and "he did nothing." One of her powerful Hollywood clients arranged for her to be seen by a different top Los Angeles neurologist. After meeting with Byrdie, this physician immediately ordered MRI and CT brain scans.

Based on these imaging tests, the neurologist concluded she had Bell's palsy, a nerve disorder that affects facial muscles. Byrdie accepted this diagnosis and tried to focus on her normal routine, which included activities such as getting her clients nominated for Academy Awards.

Six months later her father was doing much better, while her own condition was deteriorating, with the left side of her face developing a noticeable droop. So she returned to the prominent neurologist, who did another MRI. This time he said that with some rare forms of Bell's palsy, the facial nerve is destroyed by the virus, resulting in movement loss.

Because this doctor was so highly regarded, she didn't question the diagnosis. She tried to be philosophical about her condition: "My father was in remission. I had two healthy kids. I had a husband who hadn't left me, despite how I looked. I thought, *Okay, this is just my life. This is how it's going to be.*"

Three months later Byrdie went to a Little League game in Encino, where she happened to sit next to an acquaintance who was an ear, nose, and throat specialist. He knew nothing about her ailment, but he took one look at her face and, very concerned, asked what had happened.

After hearing about her medical travails, the ENT doctor urged her to get another opinion. He recommended Dr. Derald Brackmann, a renowned expert on facial nerves at the House Clinic in Los Angeles. She made an appointment and told her husband that he didn't need to bother changing his schedule to come with her; she was certain the doctor was just going to confirm the Bell's palsy diagnosis.

When she walked into the exam room, her scans were up on the light box. Byrdie's voice wavered slightly as she recounted what happened next: "Dr. Brackmann looked at me—it's like it was yesterday but it was 2004—and with a purple Sharpie pen he circled my brain tumor."

After getting the devastating news, Byrdie was blinded by shock and outrage. She called the office of the neurologist who had misdiagnosed her with Bell's palsy. She got an answering machine and unloaded her anger into it, screaming at him about his incompetence and negligence. She never heard back from the doctor. She filed a complaint against him with the American Medical Association but decided not to sue after being advised that the case would be futile since she had survived, albeit with permanent injuries. (On the subject of lawsuits, it should be noted that it is extremely difficult to win a neurological misdiagnosis lawsuit. Even when the patient dies, legal action is challenging. Take, for example, the tragedy of Beverly White, who died in 2005 at age fifty-eight, after emergency room doctors in Mexico, Missouri, failed to recognize that she had a bleeding brain aneurysm. The radiologist who misread her scan won the malpractice suit after defense lawyers successfully argued that he should not have been expected to make a correct diagnosis because he was not qualified to recognize a bleeding brain aneurysm in a CT scan, since he was a general radiologist.)[1]

After Byrdie learned she had a brain mass, many complicated surgeries and a long recovery followed. The nonmalignant tumor (a neural ossifying hemangioma) had wreaked havoc: "Because the tumor went undiagnosed for so long, I had permanent damage to the left side of my face. I cannot lift my eyebrow or close my eye. . . . [T]he longer it was misdiagnosed, the longer it had to invade the facial nerve, which is what caused the paralysis."

When any brain tumor—even one that is benign—is ignored or misdiagnosed, it allows time for it to become a stealth invader, potentially causing serious problems such as seizures, paralysis, and nerve damage. (*Note:* I included Byrdie in a *New York Times* story I wrote about the dangers posed by nonmalignant brain tumors.)[2]

Byrdie has had multiple operations to repair nerve damage and to try to make her face appear more normal. At night, she has to put special goop all over her left eye and tape it shut. She joked about how sexy this makes her look.

I asked her what she thinks might have happened to her if she had not encountered the ENT doctor that day at the Little League game. It's clearly a question she doesn't like to ponder: "I'm scared to say. . . . The tumor would have continued to grow. I could have died because it would have become inoperable. I could have had a seizure while driving and killed someone. I don't like to think about it. It's not good, what happened to me."

As we chatted, I couldn't help thinking: *If her symptoms were dismissed, then it could happen to any woman.* After all, Byrdie was a powerful figure in the entertainment industry. This status gave her access to the best physicians—but it nevertheless did not guarantee her a good medical outcome. In a doctor's office, she was just like the rest of us: vulnerable. Despite the fact that women are more than twice as likely as men to develop a nonmalignant brain tumor, the first two neurologists she consulted did not even consider that possibility.

"Anecdotally, we often hear about women who were originally misdiagnosed, sometimes for years," Tom Halkin, spokesman for the patient advocacy nonprofit the National Brain Tumor Society, told me when I interviewed him for the *New York Times*.[3]

Byrdie's health crisis, plus fatal illnesses that took her parents and brother, led to a new career. She left Creative Artists Agency and earned a master's degree in healthcare leadership, where her thesis topic was medical misdiagnosis. She then partnered with a doctor to launch Clear Health Advisors, a business that helps clients navigate their way through complex medical problems.

"My whole business is built on the misconception that just because someone is the head of a department, does not necessarily make them 'the best,'" she said. "Given what my work is now, I know that—and I think this is really important for all people to know—had a neuroradiologist read my scans, he likely would have found the brain tumor. But because the radiologist who read my scans was a general radiologist, who also was looking at elbows and knees that day, he missed it."

And Byrdie speculated that her neurologist never actually looked at the images but instead relied on the radiologist's analysis. I asked Dr. Linda Liau, chair of the Department of Neurosurgery at the David Geffen School of Medicine at UCLA, if this is a common practice. Dr. Liau emphasized that good doctors always look at the scans themselves: "It's similar to having someone describe a picture to you as opposed to seeing the picture. I never just go by the report of the radiologist. I always have to see the actual scan."

"WHEN I SAID I COULDN'T WALK, THEY DIDN'T BELIEVE ME"

Making a diagnosis from a brain scan is not as cut-and-dried as patients might imagine, as a member of my extended family, Tina Orkin, learned when she went through a life-altering medical emergency.

I don't know what the statistical odds are of two grandmothers in one family both being misdiagnosed when they first showed signs of serious neurological problems, but, in a weird coincidence, that's what happened with Tina and me. We're related through our children, making us *machatonim*—a Yiddish word that has no English equivalent or translation.[4] Simply put, it means that Tina and her husband, Gary, have a special relationship with Stu and me because our son is married to their daughter.

Tina is without a doubt one of the most dynamic and energetic women I have ever known. When she has a goal, she is determined and focused on achieving it. She worked for many years as a nurse practitioner and also as a teacher of community parenting classes. She has done extensive volunteering, including serving as the president of the parent/teacher group at the local high school. This led to a job at a university, where she worked for several years as a liaison between the school and parents, organizing large campus events. In her big extended family, Tina frequently is the person who steps up to host holiday celebrations. She has more devoted friends than any person I know and is first in line to assist them when they are in crisis. (For example, when one of her neighbors was undergoing treatment for breast cancer, Tina took the neighbor's daughter under her wing, helping her complete all of her college applications. Before my surgery, when I couldn't drive, Tina took me to stock up on groceries. And when I was recovering, she brought over meals.) She does all this while also helping her elderly parents and babysitting for her young grandchildren.

On a pleasant June morning in 2016, Tina, then sixty, was at home alone, researching healthcare plans for Gary's accounting firm. Suddenly, something seemed off. "I will never forget that day," Tina told me as we sat at her kitchen table eighteen months later. "I felt weird, is the best way to describe it. I had some numbness in my left arm, and I felt a little dizzy. I thought that maybe I was hungry, because it was lunchtime."

She went downstairs and had something to eat. She owns a blood pressure cuff, which she used. Normally she has low blood pressure, but on that day the reading was higher than usual. She looked in a mirror for signs of facial drooping, but everything seemed fine. After a while Tina thought that whatever was going on had abated. Then, in the early afternoon, she suddenly began to feel worse.

"I felt really weird again, like my brain hurt. Not my head; it wasn't a headache," Tina recalled. Her family took her to the closest hospital in the west San Fernando Valley region of Los Angeles.

There, the emergency room doctor ordered an EKG to check Tina's heart and a CT scan of her brain. Both tests were determined to be normal. There was no neurologist present that day in the emergency department, so Tina had a virtual consultation with one via computer. That specialist assessed the CT scan and concluded that Tina was having what she called an "atypical migraine headache."

Not long after this consult, Tina needed to use the restroom—and she suddenly realized that she was not able to walk there by herself. She told the nurses that she needed assistance to get to the ladies' room, and they seemed skeptical, pointing out that Tina had not had any trouble walking when she arrived at the emergency room. "I told the nurses that now I did need help. They said, 'You're fine; you walked in.' I did walk in, but by then I could not walk, I couldn't get up. They didn't believe me," said Tina. "I knew something was very wrong."

When Tina told me this, I was shocked—shouldn't suddenly not being able to walk have been a red flag to the doctors and nurses that something dramatic was occurring? The fact that this symptom was shrugged off made me wonder if the staff thought Tina's problem was psychological in nature. It brought to mind an observation written by neurologist Dr. Gayatri Devi: "It is also essential to be cognizant of any preconceptions that we have as physicians, whether 'It's a middle-aged woman—it must be a panic attack' or 'An anxious woman? Hysterical, clearly.' Recognizing and challenging our preconceptions is necessary if we want to properly care for our patients and not violate the privilege of their trust."[5]

After several more hours it was impossible for any skeptics to deny that Tina's symptoms were getting worse; an MRI was ordered. Tina happened to be friends with a radiologist at the hospital, and she requested that he administer the test. "I felt like they had been kind of ignoring everything, and I knew he would be upfront with me," Tina explained. "Immediately after the exam, he read it on the spot. He came and told us right away that I had had an ischemic stroke. None of the other doctors there acknowledged that I had had a stroke." (About 80 percent of strokes are ischemic, in which the arteries to the brain become blocked by a clot, reducing blood flow. Other strokes are hemorrhagic, in which a blood vessel in the brain ruptures or leaks.)[6]

Tina later realized that the stroke had been unfolding the entire time she had been in the emergency department: "At one point they came in and they had me sign a ton of forms about money. I'm sure I was in the middle of the stroke when they did that."

I was confused as to why the initial CT scan given to Tina in the emergency room did not immediately pick up the stroke. "This is a very common scenario," said Dr. Tarvinder Singh, a stroke neurologist with Providence Regional Medical Center in Everett, Washington. He explained that diagnosing a stroke can be a complex process: "The primary role of a CT scan in acute stroke management is to assess for bleeding in the brain. However, the majority of strokes are of the nonbleeding variety. And most of these kinds of strokes are not obvious on the CT scan, especially when done early on after the onset of symptoms."

While an MRI scan of the brain is more sensitive and is the most widely used test to diagnose a stroke, even these scans can miss certain types of strokes, especially in the early stages, explained Dr. Singh, because some significant brain changes take time to unfold and are not immediately apparent on scans.

Also, an MRI scan cannot be performed without knowing the patient's medical history. Dr. Singh explained that patients with metal or electronic devices (such as pacemakers or implantable cardioverter defibrillators) might not be able to have emergency MRIs because of the strong magnets used in the imaging technology.

Often, when stroke patients arrive in an emergency department, they may be debilitated or aphasic (unable to talk); without a record of their medical history, it is not always possible to know if they are candidates for an MRI. Even if it is determined that they are able to have an MRI, their medical condition may make it difficult for them to lay still for the duration of the scan, especially if they are unstable, nauseous, agitated, or confused. However, Dr. Singh said, an experienced neurologist can make a diagnosis of stroke, even without doing an MRI, based on a careful analysis of a patient's signs and symptoms. Having said that, he pointed out that dizziness is one of the more challenging symptoms to assess.

A case study presented online in the blog *emDocs* discussed what happened when a thirty-eight-year-old woman arrived in the emergency department with dizziness. The doctors were perplexed in trying to figure out what was going on: "Is she having a posterior stroke [a stroke that affects the back area of the brain]? How can you evaluate this patient for a life-threatening cause of dizziness?" The authors noted that about 35 percent of posterior strokes are misdiagnosed.[7]

There can be multiple causes of dizziness, from benign to life-threatening conditions. "A careful history and exam is of utmost importance," Dr. Singh said, adding that it is essential to determine what patients mean when they say they are dizzy. "Some people use 'dizziness' to describe 'wooziness,' such as what can happen when we stand up after sitting for a long time. This type of dizziness is usually not from a stroke. For others, dizziness implies vertigo, a sensation of spinning. This sensation may be associated with nausea, vomiting, and difficulty balancing and may be indicative of a serious stroke."

While a spinning sensation sometimes can be caused by inner ear problems, it also may be a clue that something is going wrong in the brain. "When someone comes in with a sudden onset of vertigo, stroke is a possibility and the clock is ticking. We need to quickly figure out if the vertigo is an ear problem or a stroke of the posterior circulation of the brain. That is usually challenging, even for the experts," said Dr. Singh. "We hope that with a detailed history and exam, we can find clues pointing one way or the other. . . . If a patient has vertigo and ataxia [a problem with muscle coordination or movement, such as walking] or if they have any weakness, that would be a strong indication of a stroke."

Once a diagnosis of stroke is made, it is urgent for patients to be immediately evaluated for possible treatments. According to the National Stroke Association, the only FDA-approved drug for acute ischemic strokes is tissue plasminogen activator (tPA), which is given intravenously "and works by dissolving the clot and improving blood flow to the part of the brain being deprived of blood flow. tPA should be given within three hours (and up to 4.5 hours in certain eligible patients) of the time symptoms first started."[8]

The results of a large clinical trial published in 1995 concluded that treatment with intravenous tPA given within three hours of an ischemic stroke improved a patient's outcome.[9] However, as reported in the *New York Times*, in the years since that groundbreaking study, a contingent of doctors have grown skeptical about tPA, even considering the treatment to be dangerous (despite the fact that tPA is endorsed by both the American Heart Association [AHA] and the American Stroke Association). These skeptics have been spreading their message on social media, where it is reaching impressionable medical students. In a cruel instance of irony, the family of the principal investigator of the tPA clinical trial, Detroit emergency medicine physician Dr. Christopher Lewandowski, was unable to convince an emergency room doctor to administer the treatment to Dr. Lewandowski's father, who was left significantly disabled after a stroke.[10]

Dr. Singh pointed out that before intravenous tPA can be given, physicians must do a clinical exam and evaluate key pieces of patient history and diagnostic data. This initial assessment must be done quickly. It starts with determining if the patient is still within the acceptable time frame for the treatment. It also is important to know if the patient has had recent medical procedures or if he or she is on strong blood thinners, both of which could increase the chance of bleeding. A CT scan of the head is done to ensure that the patient is not having a hemorrhagic stroke. A quick glucose level is obtained to ascertain that the patient's symptoms are not from low blood sugar. Blood pressure is repeatedly measured; if high, medication is used to lower it.

After this information is obtained and the patient stabilized, a neurologist determines if the benefits of tPA outweigh the risks. If so, an informed consent is obtained from the patient or family members, and tPA is administered intravenously. The procedure takes about an hour, with the patient closely monitored in the ICU for twenty-four hours.

Patients often get very good results from tPA, with the drug minimizing brain damage. "There's no way to say for certain, but I'm pretty sure if I had gotten tPA I would not have all these problems today," Tina told me matter-of-factly. Because of the delay in her diagnosis, she missed the window of time to get the clot-busting drug.

The American Stroke Association reported in 2017 that many ischemic stroke patients are not offered tPA. According to the association, minorities, women, and residents of southeastern states that make up the Stroke Belt often do not receive tPA.[11] (The National Heart, Lung, and Blood Institute defines the Stroke Belt as eleven southeastern states where the rate of stroke is higher than in the rest of the country. Those states are Alabama, Arkansas, Georgia, Indiana, Kentucky, Louisiana, Mississippi, North and South Carolina, Tennessee, and Virginia.)[12]

Both hemorrhagic and ischemic strokes can deprive the brain of essential blood flow and can cause significant disability. There's a mantra in stroke treatment: "Time lost is brain lost." In a typical ischemic stroke, the brain ages 3.6 years for each hour patients go untreated.[13]

More than seven hundred thousand people suffer strokes each year in the United States, making stroke the leading cause of disability. Someone in the United States has a stroke every forty seconds, and every four minutes someone dies of a stroke.[14] Stroke is the fourth-leading cause of death for US women when all races are combined; it is the third-leading cause of death for African American and Latina women. (Heart disease and cancer are the first- and second-leading causes of death for all US women.)[15]

Both men and women share common stroke risk factors—including diabetes, high blood pressure, high blood cholesterol, heart disease, sickle cell disease, and being overweight—but women face additional possible risks. Nurse Chantal Goudreau, the Stroke Program coordinator at the Cleveland Clinic in Florida, explained that "stroke risk factors go up for women because in addition to the classic risk factors, there are medical conditions and certain treatments that can increase a woman's risk factors for strokes."

Ms. Goudreau said that these added risks include:

Pregnancy: About three out of ten thousand women will suffer a stroke during pregnancy. Pregnant women with very high blood pressure should be treated with safe blood pressure medication. Women who develop preeclampsia (a dangerous complication characterized by high blood pressure, excess protein in the urine, severe headaches, vision changes, and abdominal pain) have twice the risk of stroke later in life. A 2018 study found that pregnant women with infections at the time of delivery have an increased risk of stroke after giving birth.[16]

Birth control pills: Oral contraceptives double the risk of stroke for women who have high blood pressure. Ms. Goudreau emphasized that before starting birth control pills, women should be screened for high blood pressure and also should stop smoking, because that habit increases stroke risk.

Hormone replacement therapy (HRT): At one time HRT was thought to lower the risk of stroke, but some experts now believe that it actually increases the risk.

Migraine with aura: Although a very rare risk, stroke is believed to be more common in women who suffer from migraine with aura and who also have high blood pressure. Smoking increases the risk.

Atrial fibrillation (AFib): AFib is a heart rhythm disorder in which the upper chambers of the heart may beat too quickly or irregularly, making a woman five times more likely to have a stroke. According to the nonprofit advocacy group WomenHeart: The National Coalition for Women with Heart Disease, a third of women with AFib do not exhibit symptoms. Others may experience dizziness, shortness of breath, or chest pain. Medical intervention (such as medication, surgery, or implanted devices like pacemakers) and lifestyle changes (e.g., a heart-healthy diet, moderate exercise) can significantly reduce the risk of stroke for patients with AFib.[17]

Tina did not have any of these risk factors, but she has suffered from fibromyalgia and related autoimmune issues for years, which some experts believe may increase vulnerability to stroke. (Fibromyalgia, a chronic condition characterized by nerve pain, is considered a different disease category than autoimmune disease, but many women who have fibromyalgia also suffer from autoimmune problems.) There is something else in Tina's family medical history that might have alerted the emergency room doctor to the possibility of a stroke: Tina's mother suffered a hemorrhagic stroke at the age of sixty. Family history is considered a strong risk factor for stroke, although Tina later was told by her doctors that because she and her mother had different kinds of strokes, their cerebrovascular events were not linked by heredity. (Dr. Singh said that in some families where strokes are prevalent, there may be an underlying genetic cause for diseases such as high blood pressure and diabetes, which can result in increased risk for all types of strokes.)

In addition to tPA, another possible treatment option for ischemic stroke patients is a medical procedure called a thrombectomy, which allows doctors to remove a clot from the patient's brain with a small surgical tool. As reported by the *Wall Street Journal,* "The thrombectomy is beginning to transform stroke treatment. Using it, a doctor pulls clots from the brain. . . . The procedure, says Denver-area stroke specialist Dr.

Donald F. Frei, 'has the same transformative effect on treating stroke as penicillin did for infections.'"[18]

As the article pointed out, many hospitals are not equipped to perform thrombectomies, and fewer than twenty states have ambulance protocols in place to get stroke patients to thrombectomy hospitals.[19] Stroke experts say that only about 15 percent of patients who would benefit from a thrombectomy get the procedure.[20] Because thrombectomies can be administered within a twenty-four-hour window after the onset of a stroke, this treatment has the potential to offer hope for a larger group of patients than before. "We have proof that it helps—we need to build the manpower and disperse the manpower to hospitals so all of our patients have timely access to it," Dr. Singh said.

In Tina's case, once the radiologist made the correct diagnosis of stroke, her family had her taken by ambulance to the highly regarded stroke unit at Ronald Reagan UCLA Medical Center on the west side of Los Angeles, a facility that performs thrombectomies. (However, by the time Tina arrived at UCLA, her blood clot had dissolved on its own, so she did not have the procedure.)

As soon as she arrived at the stroke unit, there was a flurry of activity to stabilize her. It's hard to imagine the emotions a newly diagnosed stroke patient feels at the end of such a frightening day. The nurse helping Tina get ready for bed encouraged her to relax and to not worry about what would happen next, even placing lavender-scented cotton balls on the sheets, because the herb is thought to have soothing effects.

"She was very calming. . . . She was the best person you could have on your first night, so you didn't freak out," Tina recalled. "I thought she was great. I actually went to try to see her afterward, and I left a message for her. Out of all the nursing care I got, she made the biggest difference in how I felt; she helped me believe that I could get through this. I'll never forget what she did for me."

I asked Tina if anyone from the first hospital in the San Fernando Valley, where she was misdiagnosed, had contacted her to see how she was doing. "No one ever talked to me or apologized," she said. "I got a large bill from the ER doctor, because although the hospital is in our network, the doctor was not, which is very common. So what are you supposed to do when you're having a stroke? That bill I refused to pay."

Tina spent six weeks in the UCLA stroke rehab facility having extensive physical therapy, occupational therapy, and speech therapy. She worked hard in rehab and made significant progress. Since her return home she has continued this regimen on an almost daily basis. She was very fortunate that she did not suffer any cognitive decline, but she has ongoing serious physical challenges—her left arm and hand are nonfunctioning, and walking is difficult due to a left leg that refuses to cooperate. She also is at risk for falls, since her balance is off. She has a part-time caregiver to drive her to medical appointments and to help with tasks like cooking and grocery shopping.

Some of Tina's free time is devoted to researching advances in stroke recovery. Largely through her own efforts, she was admitted to a clinical trial at UCLA studying whether or not injecting stem cells into the brains of stroke survivors could help undo neurological damage. This study involved having a hole drilled into her skull. Only one-third of participants actually received the stem cells; she will not know until the study's conclusion if she was in that group. (Six months after having the skull procedure, Tina said she was sure she was not in the group that received stem cells because she had not noticed any changes in her overall condition.)

Meanwhile, she has been getting Botox injections into her left arm and hand, to try to unfreeze the fingers. ("My hand looks very young," she joked.) She also uses a medical device that delivers electrical impulses to her damaged nerves. She believes the Botox injections have increased her hand mobility.

Tina spends some time each week negotiating with her insurance company, which seems intent on trying to stop paying for certain treatment modalities. She refuses to give up and is buoyed by small victories, such as finding elastic waist jeans so she can dress herself and being able to push the kitchen garbage down into the pail. Throughout this whole ordeal, she has maintained a positive attitude: "I think being stubborn has helped me. I try the best I can. It's been a year and a half. But it's hard; it's really hard. The best way I can describe it is, you put in a lot of work for little increments of improvement."

At one of her appointments during her recovery, a neurologist told Tina that she needed to face reality and accept that she was not going to get any better. "I told him that he should get a job in the morgue—and that he was no longer my doctor."

She acknowledged that she doesn't hesitate to make a change if she thinks a physician is not delivering proper care: "Now if I feel someone is not a good match and it's not working, I'll say 'goodbye' and go some-where else. There are a lot of doctors out there."

Although friends urged Tina to consider legal action for her initial misdiagnosis, she decided not to because she just wanted to focus on getting better. But she said she wishes there were some kind of record of her case, so that the first doctors who concluded that she was having a migraine could learn from it: "I don't know if the emergency room doctor or the neurologist are even aware of what happened. That's one thing I wish they would know, so they could learn for another patient, so they would not make the mistake again. I feel like they pooh-poohed me. When I said I couldn't walk, they didn't believe me, and they didn't give me the care I should have had. They absolutely dismissed me."

A Johns Hopkins University study found that women experiencing a stroke are 30 percent more likely than men to be misdiagnosed in a hospital emergency room.[21] When I interviewed him for a story in the *New York Times*, neurologist Dr. David E. Newman-Toker, an associate professor of neurology at Johns Hopkins who led the study, told me that one explanation for stroke misdiagnosis is that women may present with symptoms that doctors sometimes don't correctly recognize and evaluate. But another reason for stroke misdiagnosis may be implicit bias: "The reality is that, in general, women and minorities are more likely to be misdiagnosed, pound for pound, relative to white men, because in what-ever subtle ways that are unconscious, we are more prone to dismiss them or not provide them with the most thorough or aggressive care possible. Those are things that have been very difficult, or almost impossible, to eliminate. It's unconscious and probably societally imbedded in very complex ways."[22]

"IT'S NOT *JUST* A HEADACHE"

In some ways it's not surprising (although still not excusable) that many women, such as Tina, are initially misdiagnosed with having a migraine headache, because headaches are a very common reason for people to seek medical care. Ironically, while women with other neurological ail-ments may be incorrectly diagnosed with migraines, women suffering from an actual migraine may be misdiagnosed or underdiagnosed and told they have a headache from stress or fatigue. But, as any migraine sufferer will tell you, a migraine is not like other headaches—and the cause typically is never as simple as being tired or anxious.

For centuries migraines in women were considered a symptom of hysteria or of an inability to cope, explained neurologist Dr. Jessica Ailani, director of the MedStar Georgetown Headache Center in the Washington, DC, area.

"It is now established that migraines are a serious and significant disease, an abnormality in brain functioning. It's something that warrants medical attention," said Dr. Ailani, adding that the brains of migraine sufferers may be more sensitive to environmental triggers that jump-start migraine cycles, which can include not only severe head pain but also upset stomach, vomiting, and light and sound sensitivity. The headache is often one-sided but can also hit both sides of the head with a stabbing or throbbing pain. The peak times that women typically develop migraines are in their twenties and forties, with some 60 percent of these women having significant symptoms during their periods.

Cindy McCain, the wife of the late senator John McCain, started having migraines just before she turned forty. She kept the disease secret for years, finally revealing her condition in *People* magazine in 2009, when she was fifty-four. In the interview she said that she knew her husband, who had been a prisoner of war in North Vietnam, would empathize with her suffering: "I can't imagine how unbearable that pain [of torture] must have been, but yeah, I can, because a migraine may come close."[23] Four years later, when she launched a campaign for more research and federal funding on the headache disorder, she told the *Washington Post* that her migraines could last for days or weeks, sending her to a dark room with ice on her forehead. The first of many doctors she consulted told her to go home and have a glass of wine.[24]

When a migraine is accompanied by a neurological condition called aura, there can be significant and often frightening sensory changes. In an informational video produced by MedStar Georgetown University Hospital, Dr. Ailani said that in addition to vision changes, patients "can feel tingling, or like a crawling sensation, you can get weakness on one side of the body, you can get speech changes or stuttering or it's difficult to get the right words out, or you think you're saying something but the person next to you has no idea what you're saying."[25]

Migraine is three times more common in women than in men, with some 28 million women in the United States having the headache disor-

der. (Women represent three out of four of the 37 million migraine sufferers in the United States.) According to government statistics, headache
disorders are the number one reason that people seek either outpatient or
emergency room care and are an important public health problem, particularly among women during their reproductive years.[26] It is estimated
that migraines cost the United States $78 billion each year.[27]

One neurologist, who didn't want her name used, told me: "Women
present to physicians more frequently with migraine symptoms, but they
receive an actual diagnosis of migraine less frequently. Often it's written
off as just a—quote, unquote—bad headache."

She added that for many young women, migraines increase in severity
at a time when they want to be most productive, advancing in their careers and having children: "Migraines cause women to lose valuable time,
from work, from social activity, from their families."

A 2018 report from the Society for Women's Health Research noted
the significant negative effects of migraine on women's health, with little
attention paid to "sex and gender differences in migraine . . . which can
impede advancements in migraine detection, treatment, care, and education."[28]

New York Times health columnist Jane E. Brody wrote about the migraines that she experienced from the age of eleven until she went
through menopause: "Although my migraines were not nearly as bad as
those that afflict many other people, they took a toll on my work, family
life and recreation. . . . [T]he pain was life-disrupting, forcing me to
remain as still as possible."[29]

Migraine disease can affect women not just during the headache itself,
but also before and after, in phases that are characterized as pre- and
postattack. Typically, the siege starts off with flulike symptoms, followed
by the onset of debilitating pain and impairment that can last for several
hours or days. Even after the pain subsides, sufferers may feel under the
weather and unable to function at their best for several days, a condition
sometimes described as a migraine hangover.

Some experts characterize migraine disease as a women's rights issue,
with bias in how women are diagnosed and treated. There also is a stigma
surrounding migraines, with the implication that women are somehow to
blame because of their "feminine" emotions.[30] Even with proper diagnosis and care, migraines can be debilitating, affecting every aspect of a
woman's life.

That certainly has been the experience for Katie Golden, who had her first migraine with a visual aura when she was just five years old. Over the years the headaches continued, gradually getting worse: "I couldn't figure out a rhyme or reason about when they came or why I had them. There were times when I was having two or three a month, which is pretty debilitating and hard to either keep up with school or to do your job and not use all your vacation days for sick days."

In 2011, when she was thirty, she experienced a life-changing attack. "I got a migraine attack with an aura, just like normal. It can take me two or three days to get out of the funk, but usually by the next day I can at least be a little bit more self-sufficient. This attack actually has never gone away. Now I'm thirty-six and I always have some level of head pain," Katie said.

She is now part of the category of people classified as chronic migraine sufferers. "When you're having fifteen days or more a month of migraine days, whether it's an active attack or you're recovering from one, that's when they consider you chronic. There's an estimated 4 million Americans who are chronic, and four out of five of them are women," Katie said.

When Katie's migraine disease changed from episodic to chronic, she had a good job that she enjoyed, working in commercial real estate finance. "I was the youngest vice president in my company," she said. "I had just gotten an award a few weeks before this attack happened. My company was great to me when I became sick, but that is definitely not the case for most people."

Despite the support of her bosses and coworkers, keeping up at work became a challenge: "It got so bad that I would call my team in the morning to say, 'I'll be in today, but I won't be there until noon.' Or 'I've got to work from home today; call me if you need me.' And then it went to, 'I won't see you today. I probably won't see you the rest of the week and don't even think about calling me.' I called in sick a lot as I got progressively worse. It broke my heart."

Katie said that what often happens to those with frequent migraine attacks is that they get fired or "the higher-ups decide not to fire you but they make your life very difficult, so that you basically want to leave." That was never the case in her work situation, but eventually her doctor advised her to take some time off: "I was always playing catch up. I was either working or I was asleep. It just wasn't conducive for my body and I wasn't giving myself a chance to heal. . . . [M]y doctor said I needed to stop and at least do short-term disability. I intended to go back to work. I really loved my job."

But the break from work did nothing to alleviate her condition. In 2013 she resigned and applied for Social Security Disability benefits, an eye-opening experience. Katie discovered that the Social Security Blue Book—the agency's list of what it considers to be legitimate disabling impairments (the official name is *Disability Evaluation under Social Security*)—does not include chronic headaches. Katie had heard of other women who tried for years to get disability benefits for their headache disorders, and knew that she faced an uphill battle, especially after she learned that healthcare advocates had tried unsuccessfully to change the Blue Book.

"The perception is: take an Excedrin Migraine and you'll be fine. I provided them with so much detail as to how it affects my daily life. That was really helpful. I made a nine-page response to their questions," Katie said, adding that her benefits were approved five months after she submitted her application. (Based on her experience, she recommends that anyone with a disability that is not included in the Social Security Blue Book consult with a disability support group or with a disability attorney.)

After she left her job, Katie became involved in patient advocacy, writing and moderating events for several migraine awareness groups, including serving as migraine advocacy liaison for the US Pain Foundation. In 2017 she was the recipient of the Impact Award from the Association of Migraine Disorders. She also writes articles for migraine.com, an online support community: "The goal is to connect patients so that they feel less alone."

She does these activities to give purpose to her life and to share information with other migraine sufferers. All the while, she still struggles to manage her chronic pain. I asked her what a typical day is like for her.

"I always have some level of head pain," she said. "When I wake up it's a three or a four [on the one-to-ten pain chart]. I try to be active as much as I can. I do a lot of yoga. I live in Santa Monica and I enjoy working out on the beach. Throughout the day the pain will get more intense, up to a six or seven, and I usually have to lie down and take a nap for at least an hour. Then I get up and I feel better, but not great. The pain usually kind of declines throughout the night."

Katie said she gets auras only when she's about to be pummeled by an especially brutal attack: "Now that I'm chronic I typically don't get an aura, because the pain is there all the time and my brain is firing all the time. When I do get one now, I know that the next few days are going to be hell. When I have an aura it's like, 'Oh, the world is going to an end. Let me crawl into my cave for a few days.'"

Some people get relief from a class of drugs known as triptans, which can halt migraines by increasing serotonin levels in the brain while reducing inflammation and constricting blood vessels. At one time these drugs helped Katie, but they are no longer effective against her chronic headaches. She takes preventive medications every day and also has what are called rescue drugs, which she can use when a migraine is in full force.

In addition, Katie recently started getting an experimental treatment—hospital infusions of the anesthetic Ketamine. (In recent years this medication has been abused by drug users because of its hallucinogenic effects.) Some researchers believe that Ketamine, which blocks the brain from getting sensory input, may become a migraine treatment for patients who do not respond to other medications. [31]

Also offering hope to patients like Katie is a new class of medicines called monoclonal antibodies. Clinical trials have found the treatment to be effective for many patients at targeting calcitonin gene-related peptide (CGRP), a molecule that plays a role in migraines and cluster headaches. In 2018, three new anti-CGRP medications were approved by the FDA. [32]

Neurologist Dr. Natalia Murinova, director of the headache clinic at the University of Washington in Seattle who has been involved in studies of the new treatment, compared the drug mechanism to removing oxygen from a fire to put out the flame. "The results are pretty remarkable; that's why people are really excited about it," said Dr. Murinova.

Finding the right medication for a patient can be a complex process, given that there are more than two hundred different headache disorders. "I see many women who were not correctly evaluated as having a serious condition. There is this misperception, from both male and female physicians, that 'she's emotional' or 'it's all in her head.' We see that with migraines and with other serious headache conditions," Dr. Murinova said, citing the example of one of her current patients, a young woman with severe headaches who had seen multiple doctors over ten years. She was given a variety of diagnoses, from sinus infections to psychological problems, before she made her way to the UW headache clinic. "It turned out she has a rare headache disorder called hemicrania continua and there's a specific treatment, a drug called indomethacin. When we put her on it, her headaches disappeared," said Dr. Murinova.

Patients with hemicrania continua may have persistent, severe pain on one side of the face and head, along with other possible symptoms, such as red, tearing eyes; a stuffy, runny nose; a drooping eyelid and sometimes a sweating forehead. The cause of these headaches—which are more common in women than in men—is not known. Patients who can tolerate indomethacin, a nonsteroidal anti-inflammatory medication, often get complete relief from their symptoms.[33]

But for people with other types of more common headaches, long-term use of medication may end up causing new problems. Dr. Murinova explained that medication overuse headache (formerly referred to as rebound headache; advocates prefer the term *medication adaptation headache* because the word *overuse* seems to assign blame to the patient)[34] may occur when frequently used drugs cause a secondary headache disorder.

Dr. Murinova and other researchers did a study evaluating delayed diagnosis of chronic headaches and the problem of medication overuse and concluded, "There is a strong need to improve diagnosis and therapeutic treatment of chronic migraine. We found that many patients presenting to the University of Washington headache clinic have diagnostic delay of chronic migraine and medication-overuse headache. Most of these patients have been suffering for many years and have been previously evaluated by numerous providers. We need to consider the current barriers for providers in establishing an accurate diagnosis."[35]

One component of misdiagnosis is the inadequate education the majority of doctors receive in evaluating and treating headaches. "Most doctors are not trained in headache disorders, even though about a third of patients have headaches," said Dr. Murinova. "It's not a required part of the training for a primary care physician; neither is it a requirement for neurologists. It's a subspecialty of neurology. Medical school students typically only get about two hours of education on headaches."

Dr. Murinova advises anyone suffering from headache disorders to seek out a headache specialist or to visit a well-regarded headache clinic, where doctors often can guide patients toward an accurate diagnosis and treatment plan.

At Georgetown University, part of Dr. Ailani's job is to educate fellow doctors about migraine and other headache disorders. "It's only now that you're seeing more providers who are specializing in headaches who are at academic centers, and who have a say in medical curriculum. They are able to make an impact, but it's not enough to affect the number of people who need to be educated," said Dr. Ailani, adding that the providers she educates are eager to learn about how to help patients with headaches.

Katie told me that visiting the headache clinic at Georgetown University was life-changing, finally opening the door for care that helped. "If you're seeing a general practitioner for some kind of headache disorder, they usually don't have the knowledge. You can get dismissed," Katie said. "If you go to a neurologist, often their approach is to just keep changing your medication and hoping some combination will stick. Once you get to a headache specialist, at that level, they believe you. You don't really run into bias there."

The specialized care at headache clinics care may include advice on making lifestyle changes that can advance healing. Dr. Murinova emphasized that implementing small changes can add up to long-term improvement; for example, she suggested yoga, meditation, avoiding stress, getting enough sleep, and having a nutritious diet as key steps on the road to feeling better. "We call it multimodal therapy, meaning a kind of holistic approach. . . . It's layers and layers. You have to build them up one on top of each other. We know that it takes a lot to do that once you've depleted your brain energy. Don't blame yourself; it's not your fault, it's not in your head, it's in your brain. . . . [T]here is always hope, there are treatments that work, but there is not one treatment that works for everybody."

POST-CONCUSSION SYNDROME

This same holistic approach is becoming more prevalent in treating women with long-term problems after experiencing a concussion. Brain injury expert Jill Brooks, PhD, who has a doctorate in psychology and an internship and fellowship in neuropsychology, teaches patients breathing techniques and other skills such as gentle yoga and mindfulness. She also refers patients to nutritionists for guidance on changing their diets, including eating more anti-inflammatory foods that are rich in antioxidants and omega-3s. "A lot of these treatments are considered outside the box, but many of the 'inside of the box' treatments have not worked for patients with brain injuries. When people come to me, it's usually because they've been to a lot of doctors and they haven't gotten relief," said Dr. Brooks, who became a certified yoga instructor to better help her patients.

In her New Jersey private practice, she treats many people who have what is known as post-concussion syndrome, which causes residual symptoms—such as headache, vertigo, fatigue, and trouble with concentration and memory—after a head injury. "We know that the incidence of post-concussion syndrome is higher in women than in men," said Dr. Brooks. "For years, everybody was just talking about, 'Well, maybe it's their neck, maybe it's reporting bias.' Now, what we're really starting to finally get at is that there are a lot of physiologic and neurochemical, hormonal, and/or structural changes that relate to why women have symptoms longer."

In all sports that are played by males and females, such as soccer and basketball, women have higher rates of concussion, Dr. Brooks said. She emphasized that there needs to be more funding for research on women and brain injuries. Much of the concussion research done in the past has been with male football, soccer, and hockey players.

As more girls and women have become involved in sports, the rate of brain injuries has increased—but an understanding of how women experience these injuries has not kept pace. Researchers who have studied the literature on female athletes found that sex and gender contribute to concussion prevalence, severity, and recovery.[36]

Social worker Katherine Snedaker encountered this puzzling phenomenon while working at a concussion clinic in 2013, when someone handed her a pile of folders representing the cases of fifteen kids who, for unknown reasons, couldn't seem to recover from their brain injuries. Ms. Snedaker read through the folders and was immediately struck by a curious fact: Thirteen of the affected youth were girls. As she followed these cases, the two boys eventually recovered, but the girls did not. She began to investigate why females seem to have a much harder time healing after a traumatic brain injury (TBI). After learning that almost all of the research on concussions has focused on male athletes, Ms. Snedaker was determined to do something about this. A former athlete who had suffered multiple concussions herself, Ms. Snedaker first created the website Pink

Concussions in 2013 as a format to compile all of the available research on female concussions. Eventually, Pink Concussions evolved into an influential nonprofit advocacy group working to increase awareness and research on female brain injury. The group's goal is to help female athletes, women in the military, and domestic violence and accident survivors, as well as elderly women, who are more prone to brain injuries from falls. Ms. Snedaker described women with concussions as "invisible patients with invisible injuries."

"Initially, we got pushback, but now people are no longer laughing," said Ms. Snedaker, who has participated in or organized global conferences, including the 2016 International Summit of Female Concussion and TBI at Georgetown University School of Medicine.

UCLA neurosurgery professor and brain surgery researcher Mayumi Prins, who has a doctorate in neurobiology, spoke at the first Pink Concussions conference, where she emphasized the need for more research on women. She and her colleagues have been conducting rodent studies, trying to understand the long-term consequences of so-called mild brain injuries. Among her findings is the discovery that concussed female animals suffer socially, avoiding play and interacting with others. Dr. Prins said that this finding has worrisome implications for teen girls who get concussions: "That kind of social interaction was of concern to us, because during this time period when you're developing a lot of these social skills, if you are bullied, if you are alienated, if you are excluded, that very much affects your social development as a teenage girl."

Once a teenage girl has had one concussion, she is vulnerable to brain injuries from subsequent hits. Dr. Prins said it is established that for male athletes, repeat injuries that occur close together are more devastating. There have not yet been completed studies about this on women, but Dr. Prins said that "we have to figure out what's that time interval for females versus males. If it's different, then we need different guidelines. That affects how we treat a patient."

Dr. Prins observed that gender bias sometimes gets in the way of a diagnosis: "I think that, generally speaking, women probably do experience more symptoms and at the same time are considered more emotional. Because of those things, when she complains about symptoms, sometimes a woman is told that she's just being dramatic. I would hope that if you're seeing a physician who actually knows anything about traumatic brain injury, that he or she wouldn't be that dismissive."

One persistent problem with treating concussions is that these brain injuries do not show up on routine brain scans (there is a new type of MRI method that provides better images of brain injuries, but it is not yet being used in most clinical settings).[37] Diagnosis usually is based on symptoms as reported by the patient. As in other areas of medicine, women's symptoms may be greeted with skepticism. "The real key—and probably one of the most difficult things—is finding a healthcare professional who will treat you with respect and really listen to your symptoms," said Dr. Brooks. "I think the most important thing is for people to honor their symptoms and not ignore them. Unfortunately, it's not always easy to find a healthcare provider who is skilled and knowledgeable in treating concussions."

Wall Street Journal columnist Susan Pinker wrote about the cognitive and emotional challenges she faced after being hit by a truck. In addition to broken bones, she also suffered a concussion. While her bones eventually healed, recovering from the brain injury proved to be challenging. Ms. Pinker wrote: "As I was leaving the emergency room, a staffer handed me a tip sheet written for teenage hockey players. . . . There was no information for adults, nor anything on women and girls—who are known to be at greater risk of long-term problems after a concussion. When I asked the surgeon about cognitive symptoms during a follow-up visit, he exclaimed, 'One concussion! The risk comes with more than one knock.' He added, 'You'll be fine.' But I was far from fine."[38]

Ms. Snedaker has encountered numerous women who fit into that category, never getting better and gradually seeing the quality of their lives erode. "Women call me constantly to say, 'I'm two or three or four months out, and my family thinks I'm lying, or I'm about to get fired, or my kids hate me' . . . and I tell them, 'You aren't even at the sweet spot yet. Give yourself at least six months,'" explained Ms. Snedaker, adding that these women often are distraught and she has to tell them, "You're not crazy, bad, wrong, stupid, or lazy just because you're not getting better in two weeks."

Dr. Brooks emphasized that a woman with a concussion can feel isolated and misunderstood, even by her own family members, who often don't understand what's happened to their loved one: "It's very difficult to explain to people what's going on. And if you go from acute to chronic, it's often hard for the family to continue having patience. Plenty of significant others or parents will say, 'All right, enough already, you should be better by now.' . . . Concussion has been called a silent epidemic. You can look great, but experience ongoing cognitive, emotional, or behavioral difficulties."

There is an ongoing myth that men keep their concussions hidden while women talk about theirs. Ms. Snedaker calls this way of thinking sexist, because it implies that women simply complain more, rather than actually having more serious symptoms. "I did a peer-reviewed study with Clemson University," she said, "and we showed that with over eight hundred athletes, men hid their concussions 79 percent of the time while women hid their concussions 70 percent of the time. Compared to men, women were a little more honest, but we still had 70 percent of female athletes hiding their concussion."

In some situations, such as with intimate partner violence, where there are broken bones or other significant injuries, there may not even be awareness that a concussion has occurred, and healthcare providers may not evaluate for it. Dr. Brooks pointed out that you don't need to sustain a direct blow to the head to suffer a concussion; whiplash injuries from being pushed or thrown also can result in a traumatic brain injury.

"Domestic violence shelters don't screen for traumatic brain injury," said Ms. Snedaker. "Women in a domestic violence situation, 80 percent of the time they're hit in the head, face, or neck area—but in forty-eight hours they're in front of a judge, trying to justify why they need a restraining order. There's a lot out there that hasn't been pointed out. I don't think we need more MRI scans—we need education and understanding."

Ms. Snedaker continued that doctors should be better trained to recognize and treat women who have experienced a brain injury. For example, concussions in elderly women are frequently missed, with their symptoms being attributed to dementia or simply age. Because there's no concrete test or medication to solve the problem, "it's more about bedside manner, understanding where the client is and how to modify that client's life."

Overall, Ms. Snedaker emphasized, women with concussions need "understanding, love, compassion, and caring. That's not really the neurology model. . . . I think there's a lot we can do overall, just in bringing more heart into the process."

"YOU HAVE TO BE THE FIRST PERSON IN LINE TO TAKE CARE OF YOURSELF"

Maryland soccer player Brittni Souder experienced her first concussion during a high school track meet her senior year. As she was racing, she had an asthma attack and passed out, hitting her head on the ground. She woke up lying on the grass, having no idea how she ended up there.

"I got up and I finished the meet. It wasn't until I got in the car with my mom that I started asking weird questions, and I didn't know where my things were, and I was just really out of it," recalled Brittni. Her mother called an ambulance to take her to the hospital, where she was observed for a few hours. The doctors told her she was fine; the possibility that she had suffered a brain injury was never discussed.

In college, Brittni suffered three more concussions playing soccer. Although her trainers urged her to take time off, she pushed herself "because it was the end of our season, it was a big game, I had friends on the team, all the normal athletic things. So I came back and took a whole bunch of headers. I wasn't fully healed and went back into that game and took hit after hit after hit."

With worsening symptoms, including head pain and brain fog, Brittni saw a neurosurgeon. He said that her problems had nothing to do with brain trauma but were actually due to nerve damage in her neck from years of soccer headers. She took his advice and had two surgeries, which did nothing to alleviate her symptoms and, in fact, ended up making her feel worse.

When she returned to playing soccer in 2014, she suffered a brutal on-field collision. With six seconds left to play, Brittni and an opposing player ran toward each other at full speed and collided. Within minutes, Brittni noticed that her vision was blurry. "After that I started to have a lot of problems," she said, including terrible headaches, dizziness, nausea, and extreme fatigue, as well as sensitivity to light, noise, and heat. When she started to do things like leaving the oven on, she realized there was something wrong with her memory. Unable to function on her own, she moved back home with her parents. She stopped playing soccer and focused on trying to get better.

Dr. Prins confirmed that for some athletes, returning to play too soon after a brain injury can be risky, because "your balance is off, your reaction time is off, which puts you at increased risk for having another concussion, because you're functionally not back to normal yet."

When I talked to Brittni in 2016 she told me: "I'm twenty-four and I still live at home. I can't live by myself right now, and I'm two years out [from the last concussion]. I hold a job and I coach, and I do what I can, but it's not the same as being a normal twenty-four-year-old."

Two years later I caught up with Brittni to see how she was doing. Despite some setbacks, her situation was much improved, largely through a better understanding of how to care for herself. When we had first talked, she was coaching a community college soccer team, but the commotion and intense schedule made her symptoms worse. Now she's enjoying one-on-one and small-group private coaching for middle and high school students, while working on a master's degree in injury prevention and performance enhancement for athletes.

I asked Brittni if, looking back, she thinks her high school and college coaches contributed to her health problems. "When I was going through the season where I had three concussions, back-to-back-to-back, and I kept returning to play, I think my coaches then—I wouldn't say that they pushed me to return to play, but they definitely aided me in not being fully truthful," she said. "There was one practice that we were at and one of my coaches actually made the comment to me that I needed to figure out a way to hide my symptoms better if I wanted to be cleared to play."

After struggling with symptoms for two years, Brittni went to a specialized concussion center where the focus was on helping her achieve a healthier lifestyle. She learned the importance of getting enough rest, staying hydrated, eating a better diet, and not overscheduling herself. She now makes sure she has one quiet day each week, where she stays home and catches up on homework. "We have to give our body the proper tools to be able to heal ourselves," Brittni said.

Through her coaching and her advocacy work for Pink Concussions, Brittni wants to deliver a message to other women: "As far as the medical community has come with understanding concussions, we still have a really, really long way to go. A lot of doctors still lean toward just saying, 'It's in your head.'"

She advises women to "tell the truth; tell how you're feeling and then stand up for yourself. You have to be the first person in line to take care of yourself, because so many doctors still don't get it."

3

VOICES NOT HEARD

In April 2018, New York City officials removed from Central Park a statue of Dr. J. Marion Sims. Called the father of modern gynecology, Dr. Sims's breakthroughs in medicine were accomplished thanks to operations that he performed from 1845 to 1849 on enslaved Black women, without anesthesia. While many New Yorkers felt the statue should be destroyed, the plan (as of this writing) was to reerect it in Green-Wood Cemetery in Brooklyn, where Dr. Sims was buried in 1883.[1] Other statues of Dr. Sims remain standing in Alabama and South Carolina.

He was known for developing surgical treatments for vesicovaginal fistulas, a devastating complication of childbirth and sexual violence that remains a health problem in parts of Africa and Asia.[2] Unrepaired, these fistulas can cause women to become outcasts because of constant urinary or fecal leakage. Despite advances Dr. Sims made in gynecology, his contributions were fraught with troubling questions because his patients were women who did not have any voice in their care.[3]

Queens College historian Deirdre Cooper Owens told the *Atlantic* that Dr. Sims was able to achieve acclaim because he could easily obtain access to enslaved women and, later, poor Irish women. Reporter Sarah Zhang wrote: "The history of medicine has often been written as the history of great men. Owens wants to turn the focus from the doctors hailed as heroes to the forgotten patients."[4]

In his autobiography, Dr. Sims claimed that his patients gave him consent. Yet what choice did enslaved women have but to acquiescence to the demands of the man who owned them? We'll never know what was in his heart, whether he truly wanted to help his patients or if his aim was to elevate his own standing in medicine—or perhaps some combination of the two. What is clear is that there was an imbalance of power in the doctor/patient dynamic, with Dr. Sims having complete control over the women he treated.

Awareness of the imbalance of power that sometimes exists in medical care is part of Dr. Sims's legacy; it is a thread that has been woven into the history of gynecology, a specialty in which women have been particularly vulnerable.

FACING INFERTILITY

Growing up, Stephanie Levich knew that she and her two siblings had been adopted after an infection left her mother unable to become pregnant. Her parents were open about their efforts to have a family, and this had a big impact on Stephanie, so much so that she decided to make her life's work helping other people who were struggling to have children. She eventually started her own business, Family Match Consulting, which finds egg donors and surrogates for prospective parents. When she was thirty, Stephanie and her husband decided it was time to start their own family, never imagining that they would face the same fertility challenges as many of her clients. After trying for more than a year to conceive, Stephanie began different medical interventions, including taking fertility drugs and undergoing three cycles of intrauterine insemination. Nothing worked, and tests could not identify any reproductive problems in either Stephanie or her husband. "Our 'diagnosis' was unexplained infertility," said Stephanie, adding that over time it became increasingly challenging to attend baby showers and first birthday parties. She couldn't help wondering, *When is it going to be our turn?*

Finally, after undergoing in vitro fertilization (IVF) treatments, the couple was able to have a son and, nineteen months later, a daughter. Stephanie is grateful for the technology and doctors who made "her miracles" possible. She also knows she was fortunate to have the financial resources to pay for medical intervention, which she said is an obstacle for many couples. On average, one IVF cycle (a procedure in which mature eggs are retrieved from the ovaries, fertilized by sperm in a lab, then transferred to the uterus) can cost upward of $20,000.[5] Often, multiple IVF cycles are required, and insurance typically does not cover the procedures. (Some nonprofit groups offer grants and scholarships to help with costs.)[6]

For years experts explained away infertility by blaming it on women's psychological problems. "It was always the woman, never the man. You were hysterical or frigid," said Margot Weinshel, a clinical social worker and nurse who teaches in the psychiatry department at NYU School of Medicine, part of NYU Langone Health.

It is now well established that infertility has physical causes in both men and women—but knowing this does nothing to alleviate the desperation that many women feel while trying in vain to have a baby. Ms. Weinshel—who herself struggled for years with infertility before finally having a daughter—said that the intense desire to become pregnant is "all-consuming . . . you feel devastated and defective and worthless. It really takes over."

Many women blame themselves when they can't get pregnant, especially if they delayed starting a family to focus on their career. "There's still the myth in the general population that it's the woman's fault," Ms. Weinshel said, with women being told by family members that they just need to relax or take a vacation. "And everybody has an anecdote about knowing someone who adopted a child and then got pregnant. This is one of the most painful comments infertile couples get." (There's no truth to the myth—the rate of achieving pregnancy after adoption is the same for couples who don't adopt.)[7]

The medical burden of trying to become pregnant falls mostly on the woman, in the form of numerous medical appointments, tests, treatments with severe side effects, and multiple procedures. "It's very time-consuming and physically grueling," said Ms. Weinshel, adding that the process takes an emotional toll. "When I was going through infertility, it was not talked about much. I felt very lonely. Now, there are a number of therapists who specialize in reproductive health. It's much easier to not feel so isolated."

A study of American women dealing with infertility found that their stress level was as great as patients with cancer or cardiac problems.[8] About 10 percent of American women are infertile, according to the CDC.[9] With such high numbers, it's not surprising that infertility is a big business, with vulnerable, desperate women sometimes being taken advantage of by unscrupulous companies promoting false science that raises hopes without achieving results. [10]

African American women are more likely to struggle with infertility, yet less likely to receive treatment. And society continues to frame infertility as a problem of older white women. [11] One study of fertility clinics found that advertisements usually feature only photographs of white babies. [12] Michelle Obama was applauded for sharing her struggles with infertility in her 2018 memoir, *Becoming*. In the book she revealed that she became pregnant with both Sasha and Malia thanks to IVF. Rev. Dr. Stacey L. Edwards-Dunn, founder of the support organization Fertility for Colored Girls, told the *Atlantic* that Mrs. Obama's disclosure gives hope to Black women dealing with infertility: "So many black women live in silence and in shame." [13]

There are a number of causes of infertility in women, including pelvic inflammatory disease, scar tissue, infections, and chronic health conditions. More than half of infertility issues in women are due to a largely misunderstood condition called polycystic ovary syndrome (PCOS), an endocrine and metabolic disorder with reproductive and emotional repercussions. As with other health conditions that strike only women, PCOS is underdiagnosed, undertreated, and underfunded. [14] Despite the fact that an estimated 5 million American women and teen girls have PCOS, fewer than half have been correctly diagnosed. [15] Over time, the incurable condition can lead to heart disease, type 2 diabetes, and endometrial cancer. [16] Women with PCOS also have double the risk of developing nonalcoholic fatty liver disease, which may result in a liver transplant and cardiovascular complications. [17]

"Many women have been told it's all in their head, or that if they would just lose weight the problem would go away," said Sasha Ottey, founder and executive director of the advocacy group PCOS Challenge: The National Polycystic Ovary Syndrome Association. She added that she cannot think of an equally insidious condition in men that is given so little attention.

"The tool box is so limited for managing PCOS," said Ms. Ottey, a research microbiologist who was diagnosed with the condition when she was in her twenties. She said that PCOS can be emotionally devastating for teen girls and young women, with embarrassing symptoms such as rapid weight gain, scalp hair loss, acne, and hair growth on the face. PCOS patients may become agoraphobic, not wanting to interact with others, and suicide attempts are seven times higher among women with PCOS.[18] "We get distress calls from parents of girls who drop out of school because they are bullied and called names like 'wolf-girl.' This is the reality for many girls who have PCOS," said Ms. Ottey, adding that women often have debilitating symptoms for decades without getting a diagnosis or effective treatment.

Thanks to efforts by Ms. Ottey and PCOS Challenge, in December 2017 the US Senate passed a resolution to raise awareness and increase education, research, and treatment options. In a statement about the act, Ms. Ottey called it an important first step: "Despite being the most common endocrine [hormone] disorder in women, PCOS is one of the most underserved areas of health."[19]

AT RISK: PREGNANT WOMEN

In her stunning and beautiful memoir *In Shock: My Journey from Death to Recovery and the Redemptive Power of Hope*, critical care physician Dr. Rana Awdish wrote about her vulnerability when she was pregnant and became desperately ill. After losing her baby and nearly dying from a very rare and usually fatal condition, Dr. Awdish was too weak to advocate for herself. At one especially low point in the ICU, when she was in grave danger, she was alarmed to hear a resident order a medication that she knew (and that she knew *he* knew) would damage her kidneys. Later, when she asked the resident why he took that action, he clumsily explained that he had not wanted to rock the boat and question the instructions of the attending physician.[20]

After a long recovery with intervals of nearly fatal complications, Dr. Awdish finally returned to work; she discovered that the months she spent as a patient had turned her into a much different kind of doctor. On her first day back at work, she led morning rounds, where one heart-wrenching case was a pregnant woman near death. As Dr. Awdish listened to a resident recite the details of the patient's decline, she realized that what was missing in the report was "any acknowledgement of the absolute shattering horror of this particular sequence of events. They didn't see her as a person. She was a case to them."[21]

Dr. Awdish learned firsthand how easy it is for a patient's voice to get lost in the whirl of tests and technology surrounding a desperately ill person. The importance of listening to women and their symptoms is especially crucial during pregnancy, when expectant and new mothers often have a heightened awareness of their bodies, especially when something goes awry. This phenomenon was the inspiration for a campaign, introduced in 2012: Stop. Look. Listen! The goal of the program is "to empower a woman's voice as an important aspect in addressing maternal health and safety. The concept is simple: 'stop' when a woman has a complaint and no longer consider her a routine obstetrical patient, 'look' and examine the patient related to her complaint and 'listen' to what she is experiencing, in her own words."[22]

The campaign, a joint project of the Robert Wood Johnson Medical School at Rutgers and the Tara Hansen Foundation, was created to honor a young wife, mother, and special education teacher who died after giving birth. In a heartbreaking video on the foundation's website, Ryan Hansen described how his life was shattered after his wife, Tara, gave birth to their first baby. The delivery was normal, but within a few hours Tara told her medical team that she was not feeling well. Her complaints seemed to fall on deaf ears, even though the new mother had symptoms that were serious enough to cause her to faint. She felt something was very wrong: "Before we left the hospital we had asked the doctor one last time, 'Would you please check and make sure Tara's okay?'"

The new family was home for thirty-six hours when Tara, feeling much sicker, said they needed to go back to the hospital. Over the next two days her condition deteriorated as a virulent infection spread throughout her body. On the video Ryan described the nightmare that ensued: "To watch the person that you love so much have to go through that and watch her just slowly become incapacitated, it's devastating. March 31, 2011—she passed away early that morning. The thought that Tara could pass away from something associated with giving birth had never crossed my mind. I learned about maternal mortality only because it happened to me."[23]

A 2015 investigation by *Consumer Reports* discovered that thousands of doctors across the United States are on medical probation—but they are not obligated to inform their patients. The article gives a horrific example of a young woman who died six days after giving birth because her obstetrician-gynecologist failed to recognize that she had a ruptured appendix, despite the fact that she had terrible pain on her side that did not abate after giving birth. The doctor, who had multiple prior instances of negligence and incompetence, was allowed to keep seeing patients, with no obligation to disclose that he was on probation. (As of 2018 this doctor still had a practice in Southern California.)[24]

At Huntington Memorial Hospital in Pasadena, another prominent obstetrician was allowed to maintain his practice despite numerous complaints that he caused severe and sometimes permanent injuries to women during childbirth. The doctor also was accused of sexual abuse and harassment.[25]

A 2017 investigation by ProPublica and NPR reported on the alarming maternal death rate in the United States, where each year seven hundred to nine hundred women die from pregnancy- or childbirth-related causes, and some sixty-five thousand nearly die—the worst record in developed countries.[26] A 2018 investigation by *USA Today* found that many of the deaths or life-changing injuries from childbirth could be avoided if doctors and nurses in maternity wards didn't ignore basic protocols: "As a result, women are left to bleed until their organs shut down. Their high blood pressure goes untreated until they suffer strokes. They die of preventable blood clots and untreated infections. Survivors can be left paralyzed or unable to have more children."[27] Another contributing factor to maternal mortality may be undetected heart problems during pregnancy and in the six weeks after giving birth. According to a 2018 study, the rate of women having heart attacks before, during, or after having their babies increased by 25 percent from 2002 to 2013.[28]

The CDC found that in the United States, the risk of pregnancy-related deaths is three to four times higher for Black women than for white women.[29] All pregnant women are at risk because they frequently are not listened to, but "black women are the least listened to and it's costing them their lives at a much higher rate" according to a maternity expert with the California Health Care Foundation.[30]

As reported by *Vogue*, after an easy pregnancy, tennis superstar Serena Williams had to have an emergency cesarean section in September 2017 when her baby's heart rate slowed dramatically during contractions. The day after giving birth, Ms. Williams began to experience shortness of breath. Because she had had life-threatening blood clots in the past, she was sure that she was struggling with a pulmonary embolism. Not wanting to worry her mother, who was in the hospital room, Ms. Williams went into the hallway and told a nurse she needed a CT scan and a blood thinner (heparin) drip. The nurse speculated that Ms. Williams was loopy from pain medication; Ms. Williams insisted that a doctor be summoned. When he appeared, he performed ultrasounds of her legs, which revealed nothing. Ms. Williams again asked for a CT scan and a heparin drip. When the CT scan finally was administered, it revealed dangerous blood clots in her lungs, which necessitated immediate intervention to save her life.[31] After multiple operations, she then spent six weeks on bed rest. "Serena had to figuratively jump up and down and scream before somebody paid any attention to her. She knew something wasn't right," Linda Goler Blount, president and CEO of the nonprofit advocacy group Black Women's Health Imperative, told me.

Not only are Black women more at risk of dying from pregnancy-related complications, but Black infants in the United States are more than twice as likely to die as white babies. A *New York Times* investigation noted that education and income "offer little protection. In fact, a black woman with an advanced degree is more likely to lose her baby than a white woman with less than an eighth-grade education."[32]

Experts who have been researching the why of these ongoing dual tragedies believe that the grim statistics may be due to the stress that many Black women face when they encounter deeply ingrained racial bias in healthcare, including having their symptoms and concerns dismissed.[33]

This same dynamic also may explain why Black women are more likely to suffer from debilitating postpartum depression. "With African American women, there's an element of institutionalized racism, and that actually cuts across socioeconomic lines, which results in microtraumas, as well as historical traumas that cause a lot of stress and can result in elevated rates of perinatal depression," said Dr. Emily Dossett, a reproductive psychiatrist and director of the Los Angeles County–USC Medical Center's Women's Mental Health Program. While the overall rate of postpartum depression in the United States is 15 percent to 20 percent, for Latina and African American women, the rate is closer to 40 percent.[34] (Although it is called *postpartum depression*, Dr. Dossett explained that this serious disorder sometimes starts in the third trimester of pregnancy and continues after childbirth.)

In 2016 the US Preventive Services Task Force recommended depression screening for all pregnant and postpartum patients. But Dr. Dossett pointed out that there are not enough treatment options to meet patients' needs. "If we detect a woman with depression, unless she has insurance that's going to cover her to get mental healthcare, you're sort of left holding the bag. It's like asking an OB/GYN to screen for diabetes, and you find out somebody's positive—and then you say, 'Well, good luck with that,'" said Dr. Dossett.

Some women and their loved ones don't recognize the red flags for postpartum depression, which include anxiety, agitation, obsessive thoughts, insomnia, and a loss of appetite. And when new mothers seek help for these symptoms, they may be told that they just need to relax. "I do think women's health needs are often minimized: 'Oh, maybe you should just go get a massage, or you need a girls' night out.' Women get a lot of that, particularly with things like postpartum depression. It's not really that they're told it's all in their head—they're told that they don't have anything wrong with them," said Dr. Dossett.

One factor that may play a role in postpartum depression is a delivery by cesarean section. An analysis of existing studies on the topic done by researchers in China found that both scheduled and emergency C-sections increase the risk of postpartum depression.[35] This is worth noting due to how many women in the United States end up having a surgical birth. While C-section sometimes is necessary to save the life of the baby or mother, of course, experts estimate that almost half of the C-sections performed in the United States are not required and pose added risks to the mother and her child.[36]

THE DISEASE THAT WHISPERS

Stanford professor Dr. Donald A. Barr, MD, PhD, wrote an essay about the importance of listening to patients and how crucial it is to make this lesson part of the curriculum in medical schools: "When teaching my students about what goes into a good doctor-patient interaction, I tell them about the studies that show how quickly doctors interrupt their patients. Male physicians especially, I tell them, are notorious for stopping the patient mid-sentence to redirect the discussion. In one study that I came across, female primary care physicians waited an average of 3 minutes before interrupting the patient to redirect the discussion toward issues more relevant to diagnosis. Male physicians waited an average of 47 seconds."[37]

Part of listening to patients is paying close attention and "hearing" their symptoms, without rushing to judgment. For years, women with vague signs indicative of ovarian cancer were dismissed. Obstetrician-gynecologist Dr. Barbara Goff, director of the Division of Gynecologic Oncology at the University of Washington, who has done extensive research on this topic, told me that while there still is no definitive screening test for early ovarian cancer, making it a challenging disease to diagnose, there are clues that doctors often do not appreciate. Certain patterns of symptoms—including bloating, increased abdominal size, feeling full quickly, difficulty eating, and pelvic pain—are ten times more likely in women with ovarian cancer.[38] "Physicians often blow these symptoms off," said Dr. Goff. "Misdiagnosis in this country is actually very common. We surveyed seventeen hundred women and found that a third of those women were given a prescription medication for another condition before being diagnosed with ovarian cancer. Physicians just weren't aware that these symptoms were associated with ovarian cancer."

Dr. Goff and her colleagues also found that women with malignant masses typically had more severe and frequent symptoms than women with benign masses, and that these symptoms warranted further diagnostic investigation.[39] The work done by Dr. Goff and her colleagues led the Ovarian Cancer Research Fund Alliance, the American Cancer Society, and other groups to squelch the notion that ovarian cancer was a disease without early symptoms. In a beautifully written paper examining the military language used to describe illness (e.g., patients are said to "battle disease" and the United States has "declared war on cancer"), historian Patricia Jasen wrote that the medical profession portrayed ovarian cancer as a silent killer until the end of the twentieth century: "By that point, however, an alternative metaphor was gaining ground, as ovarian cancer activists, convinced that earlier detection was possible with closer attention to early symptoms, promoted the image of a disease that 'whispers' and can be 'heard' if one knows what to listen for."[40]

THE TOLL OF ENDOMETRIOSIS

Any chronic illness, especially one that is misdiagnosed and untreated, has the power to derail a life. This is especially true in the hellish landscape populated by the millions of women with endometriosis, an insidious disease characterized by searing pain that starts at the onset of menstruation and, in most cases, gradually gets worse. This is an ailment with no conclusive cause or cure; debilitating symptoms typically are treated with multiple surgeries and medications that often have harsh side effects.

In a TED Talk, filmmaker Shannon Cohn described endometriosis as "the most common devastating disease on the planet that most people have never heard of." As a teenager she began to experience terrible pain with her periods and was told such discomfort was normal, or that she didn't have a very high tolerance for pain, or maybe she was just trying to get attention. As she grew older her symptoms changed and worsened, including nausea, bloating, fatigue, and migraines. It took thirteen years, seventeen prominent doctors, and every test imaginable before she finally was correctly diagnosed. Since then, she's had three operations, with more looming in her future.[41]

With endometriosis, it is not uncommon for women to see multiple doctors over a span of ten years before learning the cause of their misery, according to Dr. Hugh S. Taylor, chief of gynecology at Yale–New Haven Hospital in Connecticut: "This is a disease where there's all sorts of systemic manifestations that are dismissed. It's often implied that women with this disease are hysterical or that it's in their head. There is some horrible gender bias and stereotyping associated with endometriosis. It's still going on."

Across the globe, some 200 million women have endometriosis. In the United States, it's believed that one out of ten women has the disease, many of them undiagnosed.[42] As endometriosis progresses, the tissue that lines the uterus (the endometrium) can migrate to other organs, where it grows, causing serious problems and horrible pain. Endometrial tissue growths can adhere to the bladder, bowel, vulva, lungs, and other parts of the body, causing debilitating symptoms in the process.[43] About 40 percent of women who are infertile have endometriosis, with the fallopian tubes becoming blocked by adhesions.[44]

Contributing factors to endometriosis may be genetics and the widespread presence of environmental toxins known as dioxins.[45] While endometriosis is not considered an autoimmune disease, women who have the ailment are more prone to those chronic disorders, including lupus, multiple sclerosis, and rheumatoid arthritis; they also may be at higher risk for certain cancers and heart disease.[46] Women often are greeted with skepticism when they describe their ailment and are sometimes suspected of exaggerating symptoms or seeking pain pills.

"A lot of women suffer from this. . . . It happens in young women with their whole lives ahead of them. They're not doing as well in school and they're not doing as well in their early career. They're making very different life choices because they don't feel that they can engage fully. It changes their whole life trajectory, so they never reach their potential," said Dr. Taylor.

One reason for delayed diagnosis is the disparity in how the disease presents. While some women have excruciating periods, others have digestive problems or urinary tract abnormalities or autoimmune-like inflammation—or some combination of these issues. In her TED Talk, Ms. Cohn said that the information medical students learn about endometriosis "is woefully outdated. And they practice within a medical system that is ill-equipped to deal with a disease that is highly individual, complicated, and involves different specialties. . . . Why hasn't everyone heard of this disease? The answer to all of those questions lies in a perfect awful storm of lack of awareness, gender bias, uninformed doctors, fragmented care, and the undue influence of commercial interests on our healthcare system."[47]

Amy M. Miller, PhD, president and CEO of the Society for Women's Health Research, said that there still is a stigma related to talking about menstrual periods, with pain and disability often dismissed as mere female problems. Dr. Miller pointed out that many women grow up thinking they just have to live with discomfort: "If your mom, your aunt, and your sister all have pain and disability, you might think it's normal. Later on down the road, you realize it's not normal."

In her memoir *Ask Me about My Uterus: A Quest to Make Doctors Believe in Women's Pain*, science writer Abby Norman wrote about how endometriosis ruined her life even before she had a name for it.[48] In 2010 Abby was a nineteen-year-old sophomore at Sarah Lawrence College—a school she loved—when everything changed. She was taking a shower when she suddenly doubled over with an intense, stabbing pain. This was the beginning of baffling, untreated health problems. Eventually she learned she had endometriosis, but finally having a diagnosis did nothing to alleviate her misery.

Reading her gripping story, I hoped that by the end of the book Abby would have found relief. But in the final pages she was struggling with new symptoms, which led to a disturbing consult with a neurologist: "Dr. Modell was not the first doctor to imply that my symptoms were psychosomatic, but he was the first to literally say the words: 'This is all in your head.' He also did so in a way that was firmly accusatory, almost to the point of disgust."[49]

I spoke with Abby in early 2018, shortly before her book came out, and learned that her health still was spiraling downward. She had lost a scary amount of weight—she has been plagued by terrible gastrointestinal problems for years, perhaps related to a chronically inflamed appendix that her doctors never detected. When she finally convinced a skeptical surgeon to take out the toxic organ, she no doubt saved her own life.

I asked Abby what advice she would offer other women who are dealing with chronic conditions: "When I first started this journey, I would have said, 'You really have to keep going; you just have to keep fighting it.' I could tell myself the same thing. But it's easier said than done."

She tries not to dwell on what endometriosis has cost her—including a college education, her love of dance, and last but certainly not least, her relationships. In the book she recounted her first long romantic relationship, which ultimately succumbed to the many emotional and physical roadblocks of endometriosis. (For starters, the disease often makes sex excruciatingly painful.)

Abby reflected: "I think I'm always going to wonder what my life might have been like if this hadn't happened. It's a natural thing to think about, especially since I was so young. . . . I held out hope for a much longer time than was reasonable that I would go back to school and that I would pick up where I left off and that it would just be this weird thing that happened to me for a few months. It wasn't going to be this thing that completely changed my life and changed me in some irreparable way."

POWER

When Sarah Salem-Robinson was in her forties, she began to be plagued by pain and heavy bleeding from what doctors told her were benign uterine fibroids. At the time, she was working as a physician's assistant in a gynecologist's office, where she helped with surgeries. A few years later, when she had a new job working in the plastic surgery department of a Kaiser Permanente medical center in Northern California, her symptoms had worsened to the point that she realized that she herself needed uterine surgery—the sooner the better. And there was something else she knew for sure: She did not want to have a minimally invasive procedure using a medical device called a power morcellator. Instead she asked to have open abdominal surgery, but her request was denied. Without any options, and with her symptoms becoming progressively more debilitating, Sarah reluctantly agreed to have surgery done with a tool she feared. That operation, performed in 2012, triggered an ongoing nightmare for Sarah that has compromised her health, her career, her marriage, and her future.

Power morcellators represent one of the most controversial women's health issues in modern times. Years after the device was approved by the FDA, arguments still persist. Caught in the middle are women who need to have surgery for uterine fibroids (leiomyomas), benign tumors of uterine muscle. According to the NIH, 80 to 90 percent of African American women and 70 percent of white women will develop fibroids by age fifty. A national survey found that Black women develop fibroids at a younger age and have more severe pain and other symptoms that interfere with their quality of life.[50] Hundreds of thousands of American women each year undergo some form of uterine surgery.[51]

The FDA approved the first power morcellator in 1991, under the federal agency's 510(k) expedited process, which fast-tracks medical devices without any testing if the manufacturer can show that the product is akin to an already approved tool.[52] Many gynecologists initially embraced power morcellators because the devices allowed them to quickly cut up large uterine fibroids. After being inserted into small abdominal openings, the power morcellator operates sort of like an immersion blender, rapidly shredding fibroids into tiny pieces, which are then extracted through the incisions or through the vaginal canal. At the height of its use, some 50,000 to 150,000 women each year in the United States had uterine operations via power morcellation.

"It really was an effort to improve quality of life for women, by offering them this minimally invasive surgery," Dr. Goff of the University of Washington told me. "Gynecologists realized that you could do this surgery, where you would just have three or four little puncture wounds in the abdomen and you could take out these very, very large fibroids and uteruses, which would provide women with much less pain and much less risk of complications."

The heart of the controversy revolves around a question with life-altering implications: The majority of uterine fibroids are benign—but what if they're not? As the Mayo Clinic warned: "Rarely, a cancerous tumor can be mistaken for a fibroid. Taking out the tumor, especially if it's broken into little pieces to remove through a small incision, can lead to spread of the cancer."[53]

The most ominous potential complication of surgery by morcellation is that a supposedly benign uterine growth may be revealed, through postsurgery biopsy, to be something else—in the worst-case scenario, a very rare and deadly cancer called leiomyosarcoma (LMS), an aggressive malignancy of smooth muscle tissue. Many experts believe power morcellation, as well as morcellation done manually with a scalpel, of an LMS tumor upstages the cancer to stage IV; other experts say that this disease progression is inevitable no matter what kind of surgery is used to extract an LMS mass.

Differentiating a benign uterine fibroid from a malignancy before surgery is pretty much impossible to do. As noted by the advocacy nonprofit Sarcoma Foundation of America: "There are no reliable methods to diagnose a uterine LMS before surgery. It is almost always found by chance at the time of hysterectomy for what was thought to be benign fibroids. There are no specific signs or symptoms, especially in young women."[54]

Sharon Anderson, president of the Leiomyosarcoma Support & Direct Research Foundation, told me she is certain she would not be alive today if her tumors had been morcellated instead of being removed in one piece. Sharon, who lives in Northern California, considers herself lucky because in 2002, when she was forty-two years old and a county social worker for foster care and adoptions, her surgeon performed an open abdominal operation to remove uterine fibroids believed to be benign. When a biopsy revealed that the fibroids were leiomyosarcoma, she then had an open abdominal hysterectomy to remove her uterus. Despite having her tumors removed whole, within nine months the cancer had progressed to stage IV, with new tumors in her lungs and lymph nodes, requiring additional surgery.

After the surgeries, Sharon asked her doctor to test the tumors for estrogen receptors, which was not common protocol. "I put two and two together about breast cancers having estrogen receptors. I thought, *Well,*

my cancer was in my uterus; what are the odds that it contains estrogen?
Sure enough, the lab found that mine were 99 percent positive for estrogen and progesterone receptors."

Armed with that information, it took Sharon six months to convince
her healthcare provider that she needed to have her ovaries removed. The
insurance company initially denied the claim on the grounds that her
ovaries were still working. Sharon had to forcefully argue that her "working" ovaries were going to kill her because they were producing estrogen,
which was feeding her cancer and making it grow.

"They did not want to pay for that. I kept appealing," said Sharon. "I
pointed to the breast cancer research. It's science: If you have an estrogen
receptor, it means estrogen promotes the growth. Here I had functioning
ovaries promoting the growth of my tumors. It's just connecting the
dots."

Finally, the insurance company agreed to pay for the surgery. After
having the operation, Sharon asked her doctor to prescribe an aromatase
inhibitor, a class of breast cancer drug that blocks the body from making
estrogen in postmenopausal women. Sharon, who has never had chemotherapy or radiation, took the aromatase inhibitor for seven years.

"There is no cure for our cancer," said Sharon. "In other words, it just
keeps coming back and back. I'm in a fourteen-year remission. My doctors think it's the aromatase inhibitor that I took for seven years. They're
convinced, but we have no way to prove it. But they know that this is a
very aggressive disease and mine was heading that route—so what
stopped it?"

Obstetrician-gynecologist Dr. Gerald Harkins, chief of the Division of
Minimally Invasive Gynecological Surgery at Penn State Health, told me
that he has two longtime patients who were diagnosed with leiomyosarcoma more than ten years ago. "The biology of their tumors is such that
the cancer did not spread," Dr. Harkins explained. (I asked him if their
tumors were morcellated and he said no, that with both women the tumors
were removed whole.)

After she recovered, Sharon helped found the Leiomyosarcoma Support & Direct Research Foundation and a Facebook support group, which
now has several thousand members. "I'm outraged that morcellation is
still going on. We continue to have new victims joining our support
group," she said.

In addition to raising awareness about morcellation, Sharon also strives to encourage more women with leiomyosarcoma to be tested for estrogen receptors, to see if they could be helped by aromatase inhibitors: "My campaign over the years has been trying to get doctors to listen to women when they ask for receptor testing of tumors, to just do it. All they have to do is write a lab slip. . . . That can be lifesaving. Some doctors say it's not indicated in the literature. . . . [W]e are still having to convince doctors all the time to do the testing. It's like pulling teeth."

She continued: "This is such an important women's issue, because so many women have fibroids. There's not one single way to know if a uterine fibroid is benign or cancerous before surgery, because they have the exact same symptoms whether you have cancer or just a benign tumor. An MRI can't show it. An ultrasound can't show it. And when they biopsy fibroids, it's like putting a needle in a haystack and they can miss the tumor altogether. A lot of women have several fibroids, so they may miss getting the right one anyhow."

Even if no cancer is present, another potential problem caused by power morcellators is that after being sprayed throughout the abdomen, some of the tissue pieces may be left behind and can become embedded. This benign tissue can adhere to organs, causing serious problems. In addition, the blades on power morcellators have punctured organs and blood vessels.[55]

Proponents of power morcellation believe the benefits of the minimally invasive surgery make the procedure a safer and better option for the majority of women with uterine fibroids. They cite the possible complications of open abdominal surgery, including bleeding, blood clots, infections, pneumonia, longer hospital stays, and longer recovery, as well as the need to take stronger painkillers for more time, a concern amid the growing opioid crisis.

Controversy over power morcellation exploded in 2013. As extensively reported in a series of award-winning articles by the *Wall Street Journal*,[56] some gynecologists actually were aware that morcellating malignant uterine masses could be deadly, a concern that was reinforced in 2011 in a small study by South Korean researchers who found that morcellation could spread cancer cells.[57]

In 2012, researchers at Brigham and Women's Hospital in Boston published the results of a study of the electronic records of patients who had uterine surgery via power morcellation. The researchers discovered that the rate of cancerous tumors turned out to be nine times higher than the presurgery predictions of the surgeons.[58]

Despite these studies, gynecologists continued to use the devices. In some cases, while patients knew they would be having minimally invasive surgery, they were not told that the operation would be done using a power morcellator—nor were they informed about what risks that surgical tool might pose.

One of these patients was Dr. Amy J. Reed, who was a critical care specialist and anesthesiologist at Beth Israel Deaconess Medical Center in Boston (where she treated both victims and one of the bombers of the 2013 Boston Marathon attacks). Dr. Reed was mother to six young children and wife to thoracic and cardiac surgeon Dr. Hooman Noorchashm, who at the time was working at Brigham and Women's Hospital. The couple each had doctorates in immunology from the University of Pennsylvania and both taught at Harvard Medical School. Dr. Reed was forty when she had surgery to remove symptomatic uterine fibroids. She had been expecting to have an open abdominal operation, but her gynecological surgeons—who had assured her she didn't have cancer—pushed her to instead have a laparoscopic procedure. (Her doctors never told her they planned to use a power morcellator.)[59]

"Amy had her operation at Brigham and Women's Hospital on October 17, 2013, for what was assumed by some very high-level gynecologists to be benign fibroid disease," Dr. Noorchashm said when we first talked in 2017. A week after Dr. Reed's surgery, the pathology report came back with the terrible news that her uterine fibroids were, in fact, leiomyosarcoma. Dr. Noorchashm asked the surgeon who had operated on his wife if she was able to get the tumors out in one piece and learned that the masses had been morcellated, "and that this was a routine practice in gynecology and that they even had a device called a power morcellator. Up to that point, I considered morcellation an arcane practice that general surgeons had abandoned in the 1970s. I knew of it from a historic perspective. Certainly the concept that an entire surgical specialty would have a device called a power morcellator designed to systematize and mechanize the process of morcellating tumors was just shocking. It was probably somewhere around 10:00 a.m. on October 25 that it became very clear to me. The initial response that we got was: 'We're very sorry, you guys were incredibly unlucky, the risk is extremely low, one in ten thousand range.' There was no sense of urgency. It almost felt surreal to me, because, as a surgeon, I'm thinking to myself, *Gee, you guys just took a sarcoma and you emulsified it inside my wife's abdomen.*"

During Dr. Reed's surgery, a power morcellator made by the German medical device company Karl Storz sprayed cancer cells. As reported in the *Cancer Letter*, after the surgery Dr. Reed learned that dozens of nodules of uterine sarcoma had been spread and were growing throughout her abdominal cavity. [60]

Reeling from the shock of what had happened, Dr. Noorchashm was enraged that a malignant tumor had been pulverized inside his wife's body. His anger grew when he learned that one of the doctors in the 2012 study at Brigham and Women's Hospital was a member of his wife's medical team. In other words, this doctor knew there was a risk of a hidden cancer being spread by morcellation, but he did not warn Dr. Reed of this possibility. The couple also were stunned to learned that at the same time that Dr. Reed was having her surgery at Brigham, another woman was in the same hospital dying of leiomyosarcoma a year after having had morcellation surgery there. [61]

Driven by grief and outrage, Dr. Noorchashm embarked on a take-no-prisoners campaign to raise awareness about what he saw as the dangers of power morcellation and to improve the process by which the FDA approves medical devices. Dr. Noorchashm was sure that his employer, Brigham and Women's Hospital, would immediately call for a halt to power morcellation once he alerted them to the dangers of the device. But hospital authorities tried to shut down his campaign and even advised colleagues not to talk to him. His relentless efforts to sound the alarm about what he viewed as an egregious medical travesty tarnished his reputation and eventually caused him to leave his job: "I generated upwards of fifty thousand emails in a very transparent way to policy makers, academic physicians, regulators, law enforcement, the FDA." As they declared war on power morcellation, Drs. Noorchashm and Reed accepted new jobs in Philadelphia and moved there to be near family. They continued their campaign to get the surgical device banned while at the same time waging an intense battle to save Dr. Reed's life.

In December 2013 Dr. Reed filed the first adverse-event report on power morcellators with the FDA. After reviewing data on the risks of occult uterine cancers being spread by morcellation, the agency issued a safety communication in April 2014 that discouraged use of the device. When the FDA's Obstetrics and Gynecology Devices Panel met to further analyze the issue, Dr. Noorchashm, flanked by two of his children, chastised gynecological surgeons, saying they "really appear to be thinking that an iatrogenic epidemic of stage IV cancer was just discovered in December of 2013, twenty years after your device has been put on the market. . . . Who exactly do you think should have been reporting these complications back to the FDA—your patients? Well, we did, in December of 2013. And now, incredibly, you all sit here, claiming that this is fabricated, that there's a shadow of doubt as to what this is. . . . Mincing up tumors with malignant potential inside a woman's body is a massive corruption of surgical technique. The mainstay of surgical therapy of sarcomas is en bloc resection with good margins—that is basic surgery. Gynecologists have corrupted that."[62]

During the FDA hearing, proponents of power morcellation expressed concern that banning the device would harm the majority of women who need to have uterine fibroid surgery. Three years after the FDA hearing, Dr. Noorchashm was still emotional about the experience, telling me: "That really fired me up, that hearing. It was just completely disgusting that we brought this massive public hazard to women's health to light—and at the hearing there were many family members whose loved ones were lost to this—and here are these doctors, their main priority is to defend the practice of morcellation."

After the hearing, the FDA advised doctors against using power morcellators, saying that 1 in 350 women having fibroid surgery may have a hidden malignancy. In November 2014 the FDA updated its previous safety communication, putting an "Immediately in Effect" advisory on power morcellators, which would now carry a "black box" warning that uterine tissue may contain unsuspected cancer.[63]

After the FDA announcement, Dr. Reed told the *Wall Street Journal*: "I think the wording is such that no sound practitioner would use it. But there are still people who won't know who will be at the mercy of their physicians."[64]

Johnson & Johnson, the largest manufacturer of the surgical tool, withdrew its devices from the market in 2014, facing numerous lawsuits from the families of women who had died, as did other manufacturers. (Johnson & Johnson is no stranger to lawsuits from female consumers: The company has been sued by thousands of women harmed by implanted pelvic mesh used in surgery for pelvic organ prolapse, as well as by women who say their ovarian cancer is linked to longtime use of talcum powder, marketed as a feminine hygiene product.)[65]

Many gynecological practices and hospitals stopped using power morcellators, usually on the advice of their lawyers. Some gynecologists applauded the advisory warning, while other doctors expressed worries about restricting access to some types of minimally invasive surgeries. The American College of Obstetricians and Gynecologists (ACOG) put out a statement praising the FDA's steps while still expressing confidence in power morcellation as a surgical option for some women.[66]

In May 2015 the FBI reportedly began an investigation into whether manufacturers, physicians, and hospitals broke the law by not reporting events of patients being harmed during surgery with power morcellators.[67] (The outcome of the FBI examination was not made public.)

Three months later, twelve members of Congress asked the Government Accountability Office to launch an investigation into why it took federal regulators twenty years to issue warnings on power morcellation, in light of studies pointing to serious risks. The bipartisan group of representatives wrote: "Hundreds, if not thousands of women in America are dead because of a medical device. . . . [T]he FDA, the medical device industry, and many gynecologists pointed to the risk of a hidden cancer as being low, only one-in-10,000. How did they get it wrong for so long?"[68]

Drs. Reed and Noorchashm filed a civil lawsuit against doctors at Brigham and Women's Hospital and against the manufacturer of the power morcellator used in her surgery. As Dr. Noorchashm wrote on the blogging platform *Medium*: "Storz executives had specific knowledge of the deadly oncological risk of their product." Storz threatened to sue the couple for defaming the company's "good name."[69]

In 2015 Dr. Reed returned to Brigham & Women's Hospital for surgery to remove a portion of her right lung, her third recurrence of the cancer. When Drs. Reed and Noorchashm arrived at the hospital they were searched and shadowed by a hospital security guard. I asked Dr. Noorchashm why that action was taken. "They were worried about my thousands of e-mails," he said, adding that he never physically threatened any hospital employees but that he did "radically assault their ethics." The couple's attorney immediately went to court asking for a restraining order, and a judge ordered the hospital to drop the security detail.[70]

That same year, Drs. Reed and Noorchashm also began to speak out against the birth control implant Essure, which has been the subject of lawsuits from thousands of women injured and sickened by the medical device.[71] Patients and advocates argued that the nickel used to make Essure coils triggered serious inflammatory and autoimmune problems. Drs. Reed and Noorchashm wrote in the *Philadelphia Inquirer*: "We believe it should be no surprise then, that women, who were completely healthy before getting Essure, are reporting crippling systemic complications that appear very similar to inflammatory conditions in which the immune system goes haywire, like lupus or rheumatoid arthritis—hair loss, rashes, joint pain, weight gain, anemia, swelling, blood clots, migraines, unexplained, debilitating pain. Removing the Essure coils requires major abdominal surgeries, such as hysterectomies."[72] In July 2018 the FDA released a statement linking Essure to multiple health risks and serious internal injuries.[73] Bayer announced that it was pulling the device from the US market because of declining sales. This action came days before Netflix premiered the documentary *The Bleeding Edge*, which looked at the risks of medical devices, including Essure. Amy Ziering, a producer and writer of the documentary, told me that Bayer knew about the problems with Essure for years, yet failed to act. "The fact that the film catalyzed enough public pressure to make them shift course indicates how critical a strong independent press, advocacy and documentary films are in keeping corporations' behavior in check," said Ms. Ziering.

In 2016, a group of forty-six prominent gynecologists and other women's health experts sent an open letter to the FDA protesting its negative characterization of power morcellators. One of the authors, obstetrician-gynecologist Dr. William H. Parker, told Reuters Health that the federal agency's analysis of the risk associated with power morcellators was "flawed, inadequate and misleading . . . and not based on science, but rather on emotional and anecdotal information."[74]

Dr. Noorchashm took issue with the argument that his campaign is emotionally based, while acknowledging that he is, indeed, grief stricken: "It's a tragedy, not just for our family personally, but in terms of, if you actually look at who Amy was as a woman in the health care establishment in our society. The fact that someone like her could fall to this, it's absolutely infuriating, so yes, there's an element of emotion to it. However, the critique is based on scientifically sound, ethically tenable data and the reality of how the system is set up. So I would reject this notion that my critique is emotional or that I'm expressing some extreme opinions about gynecology."

Dr. Noorchashm told me that he has had e-mail communications—which he characterized as "somewhat belligerent"—with Dr. Parker: "He's been one of our most vocal opponents." Dr. Parker and other members of the Leiomyoma Morcellation Review Group wrote a commentary that rebutted the FDA's methodology and findings on laparoscopic power morcellators.[75]

Gynecologic oncologist Dr. Eva Chalas, physician director of NYU Winthrop Hospital Center for Cancer Care, was one of the authors of the commentary. Because most of her patients have either known or suspected cancer, she does not use a power morcellator. She told me that she signed the letter to the FDA in support of the surgical device because she believes it is an appropriate option for some women and that patients should have the right to decide which procedure they prefer.

"I think everybody's looking for an answer that is going to be 100 percent accurate. We don't expect that from anything else in life, but we seem to expect that from medicine," said Dr. Chalas. "A physician can only offer patients guidance and data and then patients have to decide, and they have to accept the risks of pros and cons."

Dr. Chalas emphasized that there are some patients who should never have any kind of morcellation, either manually with a scalpel or with a power morcellator: "If there's any suspicion that this is a malignancy, then they should not do it. Women over the age of fifty should not do it. Under the age of fifty, they should have a serious discussion about the pros and cons and then make an informed decision. . . . [A] woman should have a right to decide."

To this way of thinking, Dr. Noorchashm firmly believes that the practice of power morcellation is bad medicine and not ethical, going against the credo of "First, do no harm." He said that nowhere does this most basic rule of medical practice say that it's all right to put some patients at risk in order to help others. During his FDA testimony, Dr. Noorchashm said: "They're saying that this morcellation is for the benefit of the majority. I ask you, where in our country, where in this society, have we accepted the sacrifice of a minority subset of women for the benefit of the majority?"[76]

Dr. Noorchashm said that there is a disconnect in gynecologists' reluctance to do open procedures. He pointed out that for decades obstetrician-gynecologists have allowed women to have elective cesarean sections, even when the procedure is not medically indicated: "The specialty of gynecology offers women elective C-sections on nothing more than patient preference. A C-section is a sizeable incision, it's done under duress, there's a lot of bleeding, a lot of time constraint, it's a technically inelegant procedure, if you will. Obstetrician-gynecologists have no problem making a big gash and offering a C-section, and here we are in the year 2017 and they are objecting to making a four- or five-inch incision to get out a piece of tissue."

Two years after the FDA issued the black box warning on power morcellators, it muddied the issue when it approved a new contained morcellator model by Olympus called the PneumoLiner, which has an attached bag designed to capture shredded tissue. In a press release the FDA said: "Although the device is an effective tissue containment system, the FDA is requiring the manufacturer to warn patients and health care providers that PneumoLiner has not been proven to reduce the risk of spreading cancer during these procedures."[77]

When the University of North Carolina was preparing to do a clinical trial of the PneumoLiner in 2017, Dr. Noorchashm presented his worries to the school and the trial was put on hold. "Can a bag contain microscopic cancer cells? That's the issue," he told me. "Here it is again. The absurdity of a clinical trial that would propose in women, in live human beings, to see if a complication that the device causes is prevented by the same device. Just the absurdity of that notion . . . how can you possibly justify exposing Jane Doe as a clinical trial subject to the possibility of her occult cancer being spread?"

As the debate over power morcellation continued, Dr. Reed had recurring tumors throughout her body and underwent many surgeries, as well as chemotherapy, radiation, immunotherapy, and drastic experimental treatments. "Amy was one of the longest survivors. We took some very extreme measures. She lived about four years. The vast majority of these women end up succumbing to the cancer that's spread in their abdomens between twelve and twenty-four months," Dr. Noorchashm said.

Dr. Reed died on May 24, 2017, leaving behind her husband, six children, her parents, and seven siblings. She was forty-four years old. In an obituary, Dr. Daniel Talmor, chief of anesthesia, critical care, and pain medicine at Beth Israel Deaconess Medical Center, who had worked with Dr. Reed, praised the fight that she and her husband waged. "What they did benefits patients overall," Dr. Talmor said. "Who knows how many women were harmed by this device? It also sets a precedent for patients taking charge, and taking control of their futures."[78]

In December 2017 the FDA revisited the topic of power morcellation, looking at much of the research that had been published since its original warning was issued and concluding that the agency must still caution against the medical device.

Dr. Harkins of Penn State Health told me that his medical center no longer allows any doctor to use a power morcellator: "Regardless of whether or not you say you'd like to use it, you are not allowed to use it."

He explained how he now removes very large fibroids or uteruses laparoscopically, employing a contained extraction system: "Once the specimen, the myomectomy or the uterus, is removed, it's placed within a containment bag of some type, and then the umbilical incision is extended, usually to about 2.5 to 3 centimeters. The containment bag is brought up to the umbilical incision, and then you just work using a scalpel under direct visualization to remove the specimen in strips externally. It's contained within the bag the whole time."

Dr. Harkins, who performs about three hundred hysterectomies a year, said that every patient of his facing fibroid surgery now is told that it is possible that the fibroid could be malignant "and we may not know that until it's sent to pathology. So we treat it like it might be a cancer, and we put everything in a bag when we take it out. That's on every consent form that we do now."

Dr. Harkins said that what happened to Dr. Reed had a profound influence on him. "The most important thing in the Dr. Amy Reed case is that she said, 'Nobody ever told me it could have been a cancer.' That stuck with me, because we didn't say that to anybody," said Dr. Harkins. "That was a mistake. It changed the way I practice. That's something every woman needs to hear. What they do with that information, it is up to them. Dr. Reed was right to ask, 'Why didn't you tell me?'"

It's now clear that numerous women, like Dr. Reed, were simply not informed that a power morcellator would be used or what the risks of that surgical tool might be. Others, such as Sarah Salem-Robinson, were told they did not qualify for an open abdominal procedure—her concerns about power morcellators were dismissed and she did not get a vote in her own treatment plan.

FIGHTING TO STAY ALIVE

A longtime physician's assistant with a degree from Stanford University, Sarah had seen power morcellators in action—and she wanted nothing to do with them.[79] When her own uterine fibroids made it difficult for her to function, Sarah sought help from doctors at the Northern California Kaiser facility where she worked. At first, in an effort to shrink the fibroids, she was given a medication that put her into temporary menopause.

"They didn't want to schedule my surgery," said Sarah. Her gynecologist did a biopsy to rule out endometrial cancer, which she did not have. But Sarah was still worried about cancer, especially after she studied a series of ultrasounds that revealed a significant change in one of her fibroids.

"No one noticed or even mentioned to me that one of the fibroids grew. Even in the report it didn't note that one grew. Any fast growth is worrisome for malignancy. . . . When I brought it up nobody seemed to be worried," said Sarah. Despite her doctors' assurances, she feared that she did have a hidden cancer.

With worsening symptoms, it took Sarah five months to get approved for surgery. After that, another battle began. Sarah made it clear that she wanted to have an open abdominal operation in which her fibroids would be removed whole. The surgeon told her she did not qualify for an open procedure: "I told him I was worried about cancer. He just shook his head arrogantly, smiling. And he repeated, 'You don't qualify.' He would not do an open surgery. He refused to do it."

Sarah felt that she had no choice but to agree to surgery via morcellation—her pain was so great that she could no longer work, and having surgery outside of her insurance plan at Kaiser was not an option. Sarah made a final plea to the surgeon: Once the operation got under way, if anything looked out of the ordinary, would he please revert to an open abdominal procedure?

In May 2012, when she was fifty-two, Sarah underwent laparoscopic surgery with power morcellation. The surgeon had told her the operation would be completed in forty-five minutes. But it ended up taking more than five hours because of a complication: Sarah's fibroids were pushing up against the major blood vessels on the back wall of the uterus. Despite this unexpected issue, the surgeon did not honor Sarah's request to convert to an open abdominal operation.

When Sarah later found out what the doctor had done, she was horrified: "He took the chance that he could have nicked my great vessels and I could have hemorrhaged and bled out and died, just so he could use his morcellator. . . . By being in there for over five hours, I also was at risk for a deep vein thrombosis. . . . He took a lot of risks with me. He felt good afterwards. He boasted to my husband about how he was able to do it. And that everything was fine. Two weeks later I got a phone call. He told me that he got back the pathology report. They said it was leiomyosarcoma. I said, 'What!? But you morcellated me!' He said, 'Well, I wouldn't have morcellated you if I knew you had a malignancy.' He never apologized."

When Sarah insisted on being sent the pathology report, the surgeon told her he would let her see it only if she promised not to overreact. As she recovered from the surgery, Sarah fought to get appropriate treatment for her cancer. She met with an oncological surgeon at Kaiser who claimed that the morcellation procedure had cured her. Sarah showed him articles explaining how, rather than "curing" her, the procedure had likely upstaged her cancer. She also showed him expert opinions that women with LMS need to be treated at a specialized sarcoma center. She then had what she described as a confrontational e-mail exchange with this doctor, whom she felt was trying to put her in her place for advocating for herself. When she complained about this exchange through official Kaiser quality control channels, she said the e-mail exchange with the surgeon mysteriously disappeared from her online medical record.

Sarah's request to be sent to a sarcoma medical center was initially denied, even though there were no sarcoma specialists at her Kaiser facility. So Sarah decided to pay for a consultation with one of the nation's top experts herself. (Kaiser eventually did reimburse her for the consult, but Sarah said the company refused to pay for the sarcoma expert's recommended treatment.)

Sarah flew to New York City for a consult with Dr. Martee Hensley, a renowned sarcoma oncologist at Memorial Sloan Kettering Cancer Center. Dr. Hensley recommended that Sarah have her cervix and ovaries removed at Memorial Sloan Kettering and also have biopsies of anything that looked suspicious in the abdominal cavity. Because her tumors tested positive for estrogen, Dr. Hensley also recommended that Sarah start taking an aromatase inhibitor. Sarah had those procedures at Memorial Sloan Kettering; later, she had another operation at Stanford University (by then she had changed insurance plans) to remove a malignant mass embedded in the wall of her pelvis.

After taking legal action against Kaiser, Sarah received a small settlement. She has channeled her anger into being a women's health advocate. "My whole purpose is to spread awareness," she said.

Sarah's ongoing health crisis took a toll on her thirty-one-year marriage. When we first talked in 2017, she and her husband had recently separated. "Before all this happened, I was healthy," she said. "We were both very active. It completely changed the dynamic. There's so much that I can't do. It was a big part of it."

Sarah told me that women still are being morcellated at Kaiser and that one woman, who had the procedure in 2016 and subsequently learned she had LMS, recently joined her support group.

I asked a Kaiser spokesperson what the company's current policy is on power morcellation and received a statement in early 2018, which read in part:

> In line with the FDA's latest safety communication on the use of laparoscopic power morcellators, Kaiser Permanente physicians carefully consider when to use this device. We always take into consideration the risks of the procedure and risks of available alternatives.
>
> Kaiser Permanente is committed to providing safe, high-quality care for women. We continually evaluate the latest evidence and treatment protocols and use that data to help women make educated decisions in the best interest of their own health. As part of our approach, we treat the needs of our patients individually, through joint decision making between patient and physician. . . . Given the well-documented benefits of minimally invasive surgery compared with open surgery, and the rarity of uterine sarcomas, we still maintain access to the option for a small group of patients in whom it may be acceptable.

Groundbreaking research by gynecologists at Yale University, published in March 2018 in the journal *Obstetrics & Gynecology* (known as the *Green Journal*) found that one in fifty women undergoing uterine surgery for conditions that were presumed to be benign actually had hidden cancers that doctors were not aware of before surgery. For women over fifty-five, the risk was even greater.[80]

In October 2018 Dr. Noorchashm launched a citizen petition urging the government to ban uncontained power morcellation. (*Uncontained* means that the surgery was done without a bag to capture shredded tissue.) As patients and healthcare practitioners signed the petition, many left comments about their experiences with the surgical tool. Dr. Stephen Hunt, an interventional oncologist at the University of Pennsylvania, wrote of treating a patient who had stage IV cancer after surgery with an uncontained power morcellator. Dr. Hunt said that such morcellation places patients at grave risk of "a death sentence of widely disseminated cancer. . . . [T]his technology is unsafe and should not be used in the modern era of medicine."[81]

In November 2018 the FDA announced new plans to create a better safety net for medical devices, including steps to improve how medical devices are reviewed and approved. As part of this action, the agency will focus on "device therapies that are unique to women, such as treatment of uterine fibroids, pelvic floor disorder, female sterilization and long-acting reversible contraception."[82] The FDA announcement came as the International Consortium of Investigative Journalists published a scathing investigation of medical devices "approved too quickly by American authorities, and troublesome ones not pulled from hospital shelves fast enough."[83]

I asked documentary filmmaker Amy Ziering if she was optimistic about the FDA's action. "No," Ms. Ziering said. "I am worried these changes are just superficial PR moves. These [medical device] companies are tremendously powerful and canny and there is no political will at the moment to truly hold them accountable. Patients need to be their own best watchdogs, unfortunately, and I don't see that changing anytime soon."

When I recently heard from Sarah, she was recovering from yet another surgery to remove twelve new malignant tumors. She told me that she has been in an ongoing struggle with many operations and other procedures, as well as chemotherapy and immunotherapy treatments, all the result of having been morcellated. In an e-mail, Sarah wrote: "I am fighting this to stay alive, but in my mind I know it may likely be a struggle I cannot win."

4

HEARTFELT

During the final season of the Freeform channel television show *The Fosters*, one of the lead characters, Stef (Teri Polo) began to experience intermittent shortness of breath. In an episode that aired in February 2018, a terrified Stef woke up her wife Lena (Sherri Saum) in the middle of the night, saying, "I can't breathe." Lena asked her what she should do, and Stef answered, "Hold me." When I heard this, I yelled at the television, "Call 911! Stef is having a heart attack!"

As was later revealed, I was wrong—Stef actually was having an anxiety attack. Over the course of its five-year run, *The Fosters* won acclaim for episodes about the challenges facing foster children, surviving sexual abuse, breast cancer, drug addiction, school violence, and the plight of Dreamers, to name but a few topics. Along the way, there were many fine teachable moments, and despite my initial outburst, this story line was no exception. In a moving scene, Stef's mother, Sharon (Annie Potts), helped her through a particularly brutal panic siege. When Stef asked her mom how she knew what to do, Sharon revealed that she also had suffered from anxiety when she was in her early forties. Stef asked, "Do you think it might have something to do with being in perimenopause?" Sharon's answer: "I'm sure it does. Back then they just thought you were nuts."[1]

As nicely as this story arc was handled, bringing awareness to the very real problem of panic disorders in women, I nevertheless wished that the show's writers had instead decided to afflict Stef with cardiac disease—it would have been an opportunity to tell the audience, mostly teen girls and young women, that heart disease is the number one killer of American women.[2] Also, since *The Fosters* had several Latina and Black female characters, it would have been great if there had been a way to get across the message that Latinas are at increased risk for cardiovascular disease,[3] as are African American women.[4] Or perhaps if the show had continued for one more season, we might have found out that Stef's emotional stress increased her risk of developing cardiac disease.[5]

In a dangerous twisting of that fact, when a woman is having a heart attack, it's all too common for her to be perceived in an emergency room as someone who simply is anxious. Despite a growing body of research on women's heart disease, problems with clinical care persist. A study by British researchers at the University of Leeds found that women have a 50 percent higher chance of being misdiagnosed during a heart attack. Dr. Chris Gale, an associate professor of cardiovascular health sciences at the university who worked on the study, said, "This research clearly shows that women are at higher risk of being misdiagnosed following a heart attack than men. . . . We need to work harder to shift the perception that heart attacks only affect a certain type of person."[6]

That point was driven home in another television show that aired during the same month that *The Fosters* panic attack story line was taking place. In early 2018 the long-running ABC program *Grey's Anatomy* had its formidable character Dr. Miranda Bailey (Chandra Wilson), chief of surgery at Grey Sloan Memorial Hospital, enter the ER of another Seattle hospital and declare: "I believe that I am having a heart attack."[7]

The episode was a master class in how a woman (especially a Black woman) may be treated—or, in this case, mistreated—when her cardiac symptoms are dismissed. Despite her status as a highly regarded general surgeon, Dr. Bailey found herself in the vulnerable and frustrating position of not having her voice heard. Dr. Maxwell, the hospital's chief of cardiology, looked over Dr. Bailey's initial test results and announced: "My clinical judgment tells me you're all good. . . . [A]ny big stressors in your life lately—any big changes?"

To which Dr. Bailey responded: "Do not go down that road with me."

"What road?" he asked.

"The road where a woman shows up in the ER with physical symptoms and you decide that it must be that she's not able to handle all her feelings. No, this is not about anxiety. . . . Apparently your teachers didn't get the memo that women's heart attacks don't manifest the way they do in men. They're not all chest clutching, vomiting, help, my arm is numb, boom, floor drop. . . . Look, just give me a cardiac stress test, Dr. Maxwell."

Dr. Maxwell refused her that test (and, in a subtle nod to the lack of respect sometimes given to female physicians, he addressed her as "Miranda" instead of "Doctor"). After she demanded a second opinion, the young man who popped in to offer one turned out to be a psychiatrist eager to dissect her home life. Dr. Bailey calmly and clearly laid out what was at stake: "Doctor, with all due respect to your field of medicine, I need you to understand that with every second we waste, I'm losing heart muscle. My vessels are constricting, my heart is being damaged. . . . Sixty-three percent of women who die suddenly from coronary heart disease had no previous symptoms and women of color are at a far greater risk."[8]

The writer of the episode, Elisabeth R. Finch, told me that when there was an initial discussion at the beginning of the 2017–2018 season about giving Dr. Bailey a heart attack she immediately "jumped up and said, 'I want to do it.' When we talked about doing this episode, one of the things that we were really interested in exploring was how challenging it sometimes can be for a woman to be heard in a medical setting."

Elisabeth had a personal attachment to writing a story of misdiagnosis, because she lived it when a prominent orthopedic surgeon brushed aside her chronic back pain with "jokes" like "neurotic Jewish women are my specialty." In a moving piece for *Elle* magazine, Elisabeth wrote that the doctor characterized her as impatient and emotional: "It never occurred to me that being 'female' was perhaps the most dangerous label of all."[9]

The doctor's dismissal of Elisabeth's symptoms was as dramatic and heart-wrenching as any story line on *Grey's Anatomy*. When she received a diagnosis from another doctor, she was stunned to learn that she had a rare form of bone cancer, which had spread. Since then, she has devoted countless hours trying to keep the cancer in check, including clinical trials, experimental treatments, and chemotherapy.

Elisabeth's own story added extra meaning to the plight she created for Dr. Bailey in the heart attack episode: "Throughout the course of the history of our show, Dr. Bailey is so strong and so powerful and so articulate and so passionate and so successful in achieving anything it is that she needs or wants. To see her in a setting where she is not able to get the care she needs is something that I found really impactful."

She continued, "Gender bias in medicine in general is bad—the statistics are pretty staggering—but when we get into issues of women of color, it's even more so. I just wanted to take the opportunity to highlight that as much as possible."

Right about now you might be wondering why television shows even matter in a discussion of women and heart disease. The answer is simple: The majority of teenage girls and young women don't read newspapers or serious magazines, and certainly not medical journals. Unless the information reaches them on one of their electronic devices, most will never be aware that there's a distinct possibility they may one day face cardiac problems.[10]

"We learn a lot from entertainment and from TV. The typical Hollywood heart attack was always an overweight man, or a man having an affair; he would get blue in the face, clutch his chest and fall to the ground. . . . [I]t's only been in the last couple of years that we've seen a woman have a heart attack on screen," said cardiologist Dr. Suzanne Steinbaum, director of Women & Heart Health at Lenox Hill Hospital in New York City.

As a national spokesperson for the American Heart Association's Go Red for Women campaign, Dr. Steinbaum has been part of an ongoing attempt to raise awareness about women's cardiac risks. The AHA launched Go Red in 2004 in an effort to change the grim statistic of five hundred thousand American women dying each year from heart issues. A central focus has been trying to correct the misconception that heart disease is a male problem; because most cardiac research has been conducted on men, this has led to an "oversimplified, distorted view of heart disease and risk, which has worked to the detriment of women. Because women have been largely ignored as a specific group, their awareness of their risk of this often-preventable disease has suffered."[11]

Among the cardiac symptoms that women may experience—and which they may not recognize as heart related—are pressure or discomfort in the chest and pain in the arms, back, neck, jaw or stomach; as well as shortness of breath, fatigue, nausea, vomiting, lightheadedness or sweating.[12] There is a lack of awareness of risks for heart disease, including high blood pressure, high LDL and overall cholesterol, menopause, smoking, diabetes, being overweight, not exercising, poor diet, heavy alcohol use, and certain pregnancy complications. Other risk factors are stress and depression, more so for women than men. Family history of heart disease also plays a significant role. [13]

In 2012 television celebrity Rosie O'Donnell waited a day to seek medical help, despite experiencing pain, nausea, clammy skin, and vomiting. She looked up heart attack symptoms online and then took an aspirin, but, as she later wrote on her blog, she did not call 911. When she saw a cardiologist the next day, she was given an EKG that revealed that she needed a stent in her left anterior descending artery, which was almost completely blocked, a type of heart attack called "the widow-maker." Ms. O'Donnell, knowing how lucky she was to have survived, implored her readers to "know the symptoms. . . . [L]isten to the voice inside, the one we all so easily ignore. CALL 911." [14] To help raise awareness, she created an acronym to alert women to possible heart attack symptoms: HEPPP, which stands for hot, exhausted, pain, pale, puke.

Not only do many women not recognize symptoms that are red flags for cardiac distress, even some physicians aren't able to correctly evaluate the signs. In one study, when symptomatic women under the age of fifty-five saw their primary care doctors prior to having a heart attack, 56 percent were told that their symptoms were not cardiac related, even when there was a family history of heart disease. The lead author of the study noted that young women with heart disease have double the risk of dying in the hospital than do similarly aged men. [15] In another study, researchers at the Yale School of Public Health reported that young women presenting with heart attack symptoms were likely to have their concerns dismissed by doctors, despite the fact that all of these women had cardiac risk factors. [16]

"More times than I can tell you, women with cardiac symptoms have said to me that they were told by doctors that they're anxious, they're depressed. . . . [T]hat has been the most common thing I hear in my office," said Dr. Steinbaum. "These women tell me, 'I know it's not all in my head.' I hear it all the time. The other issue is that a lot of women look good on the outside, but that's not really what's going on, on the inside. They might be thin and well-dressed, with lipstick and makeup—but they can still have heart disease."

When Dr. Steinbaum began her cardiology fellowship in 1998 at Beth Israel Medical Center in New York City, there were only a handful of female doctors in the program: "I was there before there really was such a thing as 'women and heart disease.'"

As a second-year resident, she witnessed a fifty-three-year-old woman being wheeled into the emergency room. It was a case that has stayed with Dr. Steinbaum and inspired her to advocate for women: "She was very uncomfortable—sweating, nauseous, very sick—and they put her in the corner with a diagnosis of gastroenteritis. I watched her have a heart attack in the emergency room. I was in my training, and doctors who I really respected let this happen. And it wasn't the first time. . . . One thing I learned in my fellowship is 'time is muscle.' That's what the head of our program used to say. The quicker you can diagnose, the sooner you can save their heart. What happened to that woman was such a motivating moment. I knew very clearly what I wanted to do."

"I KEPT SAYING, 'I CAN'T BREATHE'"

In 2014, when Yesenia Araujo was forty-three, she was hurrying to board a commuter train in New York City when she suddenly felt short of breath and collapsed. She was taken to an emergency room, where she was asked if she was under stress. When she assured the doctor that she was not anxious, he diagnosed her with asthma and prescribed an inhaler.

Back home, Yesenia couldn't shake the feeling that something else was going on. Instead of getting better, she felt worse. "I kept saying, I can't breathe. It felt like my chest was caving in or like an elephant was sitting on it. So they rushed me to another hospital and started doing a lot of tests. This time there was no denying that I was having a heart attack." In fact, her previous misdiagnosis may have triggered the second heart attack, because the steroids in the inhaler had escalated her cardiac crisis.

The first ER doctor who treated her did not consider her family risk—Yesenia's father died from a massive heart attack. Even Yesenia herself did not realize the implications of her father's heart disease; no doctor had ever discussed the seriousness of her family history with her. "I didn't realize that my father's heart disease put me at risk; I had no clue. I didn't understand what that meant. Hereditary? I thought that meant that my father left me money," she joked. "He did leave me something—he left me heart disease!"

Yesenia had a stent put in, and she now is under the care of a good cardiologist and on heart medication as well as a statin drug. "I trusted the first doctor I saw. . . . It didn't occur to him I could be having a heart attack because of my age, because I'm female, became I'm Latina. We're not put in the same category," said Yesenia. "There are a lot of women who are misdiagnosed. We're all in the same boat; we're dealing with heart issues and how people mistreat us or think it's not a big deal. But it is a big deal. And we're living proof that it can happen at any age."

Too sick to work, Yesenia became a volunteer for the advocacy organization WomenHeart. The nonprofit was founded in 1999 by three women in their forties who had heart attacks that were misdiagnosed. Nancy Loving, Jackie Markham, and Judy Mingram did not know each other and lived in different cities, but all experienced inadequate treatment for their cardiac disease. They also realized how little information was available for women dealing with heart problems. Eventually the three women teamed up to start a support group that went on to become WomenHeart, with the mission of educating and improving the lives of women with heart disease.[17]

"We have to educate ourselves to know what are our symptoms and what's going on with our bodies. I didn't know how to explain that I really couldn't breathe. I didn't realize it could be a symptom of a heart attack," Yesenia said. "And that's where the misdiagnosis comes in. We believe the doctors right away, because they're the ones who went to school for fourteen years. We just trust them when they say they'll make it all better."

During most women's routine physicals or other medical appointments, cardiac disease is rarely discussed. As reported by Harvard Health, "many women say their physicians never talk to them about coronary risk and sometimes don't even recognize the symptoms, mistaking them instead for signs of panic disorder, stress, and even hypochondria."[18]

Margo Minissian, PhD, a research scientist, cardiology nurse practitioner, and clinical lipid specialist at the Barbra Streisand Women's Heart Center in the Smidt Heart Institute at Cedars-Sinai in Los Angeles, said it's crucial to get the word "out into the community that heart disease can present in many different fashions. Essentially, any symptom above your waist could be a cardiac symptom. For many women it's shortness of breath and excessive fatigue. Sometimes women's symptoms are described as 'atypical.' In fact, they're not atypical for women, but they're atypical for the classic male Hollywood heart attack, if you will, that has been painted."

Neurologist Dr. Gayatri Devi wrote about the cardiac misdiagnosis of one of her patients: "Gender bias hinders accurate diagnosis more often than I would like, and not just with brain disorders. For example, Marjorie, a patient whom I saw for migraines, raced to the emergency room with chest pains when she was 48, worried she was experiencing a heart attack. To her relief, she was told that she was just experiencing a panic attack and should go home."[19]

This story did not have a happy ending. After having her symptoms dismissed, Marjorie collapsed and later learned she had suffered a major heart attack, which had been preceded by multiple smaller attacks and a missed diagnosis of a blood-clotting disorder. Marjorie died five years later from heart disease. Observed Dr. Devi: "I am hard put to think of a circumstance in which a 40-year-old male patient with chest pains would have been told he was having a panic attack and sent home from the hospital."[20]

"YOU'RE HAVING A PANIC ATTACK"

On a Friday morning in 2010, Becky Kranig suddenly started to feel sick. She was a busy thirty-seven-year-old wife and mother with two toddler sons. Most days she worked in her camping store, Bearcub Outfitters, in Petoskey, Michigan. On this particular morning the family was up early. One of the boys had an appointment with an allergist. Her husband, Brad, had a work meeting, and everyone was getting ready for a busy day.

Becky was brushing her teeth when she became aware that something was wrong. Brad commented, "You don't look very good." Becky replied, "I don't feel very good."

"It wasn't like a screaming pain," Becky recalled, "but it was a major discomfort; it felt like heartburn radiating through my whole chest. I didn't get heartburn very often. What is this feeling?"

Usually, if she had a cold or a virus, she could muddle through. But this was different: "I tried to finish getting ready, but I kept thinking, *You know, the way that I feel, I don't think I can take care of my kids.*"

Her husband hurried to their computer in the basement. "I was still trying to figure out what was going on," she said. "And I finally yelled down to him, 'Can you look up the symptoms for women and heart attacks?' And he said, 'I already am.' He asked me if I had any tingling feeling. I told him I was kind of tingling all over, but my adrenaline was going because I was starting to get scared. Brad said that I was extremely pale. He'd never seen me look like that, not even when I was sick. I was a bizarre shade of gray."

At that point her husband announced, "We're going to the hospital."

Before they could leave, they had to wait for a grandparent to arrive to watch the boys. "While we were waiting for my dad to come over to be with the kids, my husband told me, 'Take one of Darby's aspirins. It can't hurt anything.'"

Darby, their aging dog, was on a regimen of adult (human) aspirin and Becky swallowed one pill. Her father arrived soon after, and Brad drove Becky to the hospital, which was two miles away. From the time she first started feeling sick, about a half hour had passed.

At the hospital she was immediately given an EKG as well as blood tests to check her enzymes, which can detect heart muscle damage. All of the tests results came back normal. Becky eventually became aware that there seemed to be a consensus among the doctors and nurses that she had had a panic attack and that the appropriate course of action would be to send her home. But one member of the ER team disagreed with this assessment. He was an emergency room technician who, coincidentally, happened to be a regular customer at Becky's store.

This ER tech advised Becky to stay put because he wanted to repeat the enzyme blood test after an hour and a half. He commented that he had seen Becky in action during busy times at the store and that she had never struck him as a person who would panic.

The repeat blood test showed that her enzymes had elevated slightly, from 0 to 1.5. (The magic number for the hospital to admit a patient with suspected heart trouble was an enzyme level of 5.) The ER tech urged Becky to stay for another ninety minutes, when he would do the blood test again. This time the enzyme level was 3. When the test was repeated a forth time, the level was 5 and Becky was admitted to the cardiac unit. Additional testing confirmed that she had had a heart attack and had suffered cardiac damage.

Because Becky was a young, thin, athletic, nonsmoker, cardiac disease was not on the radar of the doctors and nurses who examined her in the emergency room. If not for the ER technician who refused to let her be released, she could have had a dire outcome.

"He really did fight for me," said Becky. "If it wasn't for him, I would have gone back home and maybe had another heart attack."

Becky had no preexisting conditions or family history of cardiac disease, but she had been on birth control pills for about fifteen years, which she believes caused her heart attack. While considered safe for most women, the estrogen in birth control pills can increase the risk of heart attack, particularly in women over thirty-five.[21]

One of the elements of Becky's case that might seem puzzling is that her first EKG was normal, leading most of the ER workers to conclude that she was not having a heart attack. But Dr. Laxmi Mehta, a noninvasive cardiologist and section director of Preventative Cardiology and Women's Cardiovascular Health at the Ohio State University Wexner Medical Center, explained that, actually, that kind of early test result is not surprising, because regardless of gender, an EKG can be normal—or only slightly abnormal—if the patient is having a mild heart attack. "An EKG is helpful in determining if it's a major heart attack, but some heart attacks can be missed based on the initial EKG, and so it is important to check serial EKGs and blood tests while also reassessing the patient's symptoms," said Dr. Mehta.

As for Becky's initial enzyme blood test, which also was normal, Dr. Mehta said that can happen when a patient first arrives at the hospital, because of the nature of the test. "The initial cardiac biomarker, troponin level, can be normal even if someone is having a major heart attack," said Dr. Mehta. "That blood test measures the levels of proteins that are released into the bloodstream when there is heart muscle damage. Within the first three to four hours it can still be normal, which is the case when the patient comes in soon after the onset of symptoms. That's why we usually will check serial biomarkers. If someone comes in with symptoms suggestive of a heart attack, we will urge them to stay even if the EKG is normal, just to make sure we're not missing 'minor' types of heart attacks."

When I told her about Becky's case, Dr. Mehta speculated that most likely one of the factors working against Becky's getting a correct diagnosis was that she was younger than most heart attack victims. "A lot of times younger women are told, 'You're having a panic attack. Just calm down,'" said Dr. Mehta, although she believes most emergency room staff now have increased awareness of possible atypical cardiac symptoms in women.

"I think it's improved with protocols that are in place. For example, most people that come into an emergency room with any symptom from the waist up to the neck are likely to have at least an EKG, depending on the nature of their symptoms," said Dr. Mehta. "Even when women come into the hospital, their atypical symptoms may be missed but that is less likely to occur if they wait long enough for the serial blood tests. Sometimes when they come in and they haven't had a heart attack but they're having the start of the atypical symptoms that precede an attack, those symptoms may be dismissed and they're sent home. We always recommend that patients follow up with their doctor, because even if they did not have a heart attack, the fact that they are having symptoms means they need further workup as an outpatient for heart artery blockages."

The National Heart, Lung, and Blood Institute says that many women delay getting help for possible cardiac symptoms "because they don't want to bother others, especially if their symptoms turn out to be a 'false alarm.' But when you're facing something as serious as a possible heart attack, it is much better to be safe than sorry."[22]

Family members also may not recognize the signs of a heart attack. And even if an ambulance is called, responders might not realize a female patient is having a cardiac event, particularly if the symptoms are different than what they've seen in the past. In 2018, researchers at George Washington University found that after a 911 call, men and women with heart attack symptoms receive very different care from emergency medical services, with women less likely to be resuscitated, given aspirin, or sped to the hospital in an ambulance using lights and sirens.[23]

For many years, heart disease was considered solely a male problem. In her groundbreaking 2002 book about women and heart disease, *Women Are Not Small Men*, cardiologist Dr. Nieca Goldberg wrote: "Until very recently, no book like this could have been written, because all of the knowledge, research, and treatments concerning heart disease were based on findings in men. For too many years, the medical establishment was ignorant of women's unique needs and physiology and looked upon women as simply 'small men.'"[24]

In a 2018 *New York Times* report, one of Dr. Goldberg's patients, Edna Haber, told the newspaper that while she has had wonderful male and female doctors, her worst medical experiences have involved male doctors who dismissed her symptoms or even screamed at her when she questioned a medical test. When she began to experience cardiac symptoms, she went to see Dr. Goldberg, medical director of the Joan H. Tisch Center for Women's Health at NYU Langone Health. Dr. Goldberg had Ms. Haber wear a heart monitor, which revealed the need for a pacemaker to correct a heart rhythm problem. Ms. Haber told the newspaper: "I do believe that had I been with a male doctor, I think he just would have put his arm around me and said, 'Listen, go home, relax, meditate, maybe take a tranquilizer,' and that would have been the end of it."[25]

It's been known for some time that women are less likely than men to survive in the aftermath of a heart attack. A startling new twist to this fact was revealed in a large 2018 study that found that female cardiac patients were more likely to die when treated in an emergency room by a male doctor. Researchers from Washington University, Harvard, and the University of Minnesota reviewed 582,000 heart attack cases treated in Florida emergency rooms over a span of nineteen years and found that when women were treated by a female doctor the survival rate was higher.[26] The researchers determined that male and female cardiac patients have similar outcomes when treated by a female physician but that "unique challenges arise when male physicians treat female patients. We further find that male physicians with more exposure to female patients and female physicians have more success treating female patients."[27]

One of the study researchers, Brad Greenwood, PhD, an associate professor of information and decision sciences at the University of Minnesota Carlson School of Management, told me that the study reinforces how important diversity is among emergency room physicians and cardiologists, two specialties that have traditionally been dominated by white men. "Within the context of the paper, we do see that as the number of female colleagues increases, the performance of male physicians improves, as well," said Dr. Greenwood. "This could be as a result of direct learning, it could be an over the shoulder tap—'Oh hey, you should look at this.' It could be learning through emulation; it could be just a general increase in awareness."

Dr. Greenwood emphasized that the takeaway from the research paper is not that women should avoid male doctors: "That's the wrong conclusion, for a couple of reasons. One, it doesn't solve the actual problem, and you don't always have that option. Second, there's such a wide disparity in performance in physicians. . . . There are male and female doctors who are amazingly good and there also are male and female doctors who don't perform as well."

He speculated that in some cases, female patients may be more comfortable advocating for themselves and communicating with a female physician, particularly if they've had experiences in which a male doctor dismissed or misread their symptoms. In an acute cardiac crisis, if a physician is not well versed in women's possible symptoms or doesn't really listen to a female patient's description of her condition, a bad outcome is inevitable. "It's critical that we keep doing more research on this subject to try and figure out exactly what's going on," said Dr. Greenwood.

Dr. Martha Gulati, chief of cardiology at the University of Arizona College of Medicine–Phoenix, said that women continue to have symptoms that get ignored or misinterpreted: "Additionally, even when they get a diagnosis of heart disease or if they've had a heart attack, if it's clear—why is it that we still treat women differently? Our national data shows that women are less likely to get guideline recommended therapy, simple things like aspirin, statins, beta blockers, ACE inhibitors. Even after a heart attack, she is less likely to get the recommended door-to-balloon time, to open up the artery as quickly as possible. Women are less likely to achieve those door-to-balloon times than are men." (Door-to-balloon time is the time between when a heart attack patient with a blocked artery arrives in the emergency room to when the artery is opened up, saving the patient's life.)

Dr. Gulati's voice rose when she discussed how women sometimes are treated in emergency rooms: "As women we should be outraged; we are consumers of healthcare and we should demand respect for ourselves and our symptoms. . . . There should be a public outcry for the differences in how we're treated compared to how men are treated. . . . If I'm having a heart attack, I want no delay. I want the guideline effective therapy given to me and I want my coronary opened up quickly. I don't have time for chitchat. I don't want somebody asking me if I'm stressed out. Of course I'm stressed out! We're all stressed out! Why do men not get asked those questions? There's something about presenting as a woman, whatever that is, that we get treated differently."

While some women have less-common symptoms, other women appear in emergency rooms with typical symptoms. "When they have a heart attack, two-thirds of women will present with crushing chest pain, shortness of breath, left arm pain, shoulder pain, the whole classic image—but even those can get missed in the emergency room. The other third might present with more atypical symptoms, not with any chest pain at all but more subtle symptoms. I agree, these might be harder for us to recognize, but we still need to be able to recognize them. But why do we miss symptoms when they're so common?" Dr. Gulati asked.

Carolyn Thomas, author of the popular blog *Heart Sisters*, recounted in her book *A Woman's Guide to Living with Heart Disease* how she experienced alarming symptoms during her morning walk, including chest pain, nausea, sweating, and "hot prickly pressure radiating down my left arm." She went to a nearby hospital emergency room and told the admitting nurse that she thought she was having a heart attack. She was given an EKG and a cardiac enzyme blood test, which came back normal, leading the ER doctor to diagnose her with acid reflux. Before she left the hospital she was scolded by a nurse, who let her know that she should not have pestered the doctor because "he does not like to be questioned." (It turned out that Carolyn had offended him after he offered his diagnosis by asking, "What about this pain down my left arm?")[28]

Despite a new regimen of Gaviscon to fight her supposed acid reflux, Carolyn continued to experience worrisome symptoms. She even traveled to celebrate her mother's eightieth birthday. By the end of the trip she was so ill she could barely make it off the plane. She later reflected that "what I've just described during that two-week nightmare now seems like a case of denial on steroids. How could I possibly have interpreted my symptoms as simple heartburn, even as they worsened day by day? I'm not a physician, but even I knew that pain down your left arm isn't a sign of acid reflux, so why did I continue to cling so dangerously to what that ER doctor had told me?"[29]

Carolyn eventually learned that she has a serious condition called microvascular heart disease (MVD), which damages small arteries of the heart. Cardiologist Dr. Stacey Rosen, a spokesperson for the AHA, said in a *New York Times* "Ask Well" column that MVD, which affects about four times as many women as men, can lead to heart attack, cardiac arrest, and death. Dr. Rosen explained that MVD "absolutely can be treated and needs to be treated. Decades ago, when we didn't understand this, we told women they didn't have heart disease and they should take Maalox or anti-anxiety medication, when in fact this was a form of ischemic heart disease that was poorly understood."[30]

A 2016 study found that women brought to a hospital after cardiac arrest may be less likely to receive lifesaving treatments, resulting in higher in-hospital mortality.[31] Lead author Dr. Luke Kim, a cardiologist at Weill Cornell Medical College in New York said that "the troublesome part of our paper is that just as with many other treatments we're still not doing as good a job with women as men. Women tend to get less immediate care when time is essential."[32]

DIAGNOSIS: DRAMA QUEEN

As a young girl growing up in the California high desert, Starr Mirza loved sports: "When I was a kid I was extremely active. Any sport that they let me play, I played. I ran track and I played softball and tennis."

The only downside was that Starr sometimes passed out while running around. And she was constantly tired, no matter how much sleep she got. Her mother and stepfather did not have much money, so they took her repeatedly to the local county hospital, where doctors could not find a cause for her fainting and fatigue.

"I can tell you that a couple of doctors—I remember them like it was an hour ago—came in and saw that I was female and just rolling their eyes and not even doing tests," she said. "They wanted to know what I had to eat; they wanted to know if I had a boyfriend; they wanted to know if I was popular or had problems at school. That would be the extent of the appointment."

This went on for years. By the time Starr was a teenager, there were several prevailing theories about what was wrong with her: She was not eating enough because she was worried about her weight; she was faking the symptoms; she just wanted to be the center of attention. One time Starr overheard a doctor tell her parents that she had Munchausen syndrome, a psychological disorder in which a person feigns serious illness. Her parents followed the doctor's advice and took Starr to several psychiatrists, none of whom could find evidence of mental illness.

"It became a big thing in my family: I was a drama queen and was doing it for attention," Starr continued. "Being female is difficult enough, especially when you're in your teen years. I wasn't suicidal, but I started to think: *I can't live like this*."

One time she passed out in PE class: "They brought a wheelchair down from the nurse's office. My mom was a cafeteria worker with the school. As they wheeled me down the hall, I remember seeing my mom and her looking at me with such disgust and telling me to get out of the wheelchair because I was embarrassing her."

Because she was constantly exhausted, Starr decided that maybe her problem was that she wasn't getting enough sleep. "I pretended that I was going to school, but I would actually park my car around the corner and sneak back in the house and take a nap under my bed," she said. "I just didn't want them to think that I was lazy. You're still hearing that they can't find anything wrong. I started to think that maybe this is all in my head. Maybe it's something that I'm creating."

Through it all, Starr tried to live the normal life of a teenager: "I didn't want to stop playing sports and hanging out with friends. I just pushed myself, and I was always so tired. My friends were sneaking out to be with their boyfriends or to go drinking—I was sneaking to find places to take naps."

After high school she moved out, eager to get away from an emotionally abusive environment. She worked two jobs, one in a pizza factory and another as a waitress, while also taking college classes. But her fainting spells continued, so she stopped going to school. After she met her boyfriend, who was in the US Air Force, she convinced herself that getting married and moving to Florida would be the fresh start she needed and that she could leave behind her health problems. But instead, when she was twenty-two, she got worse, becoming ill with bouts of pleurisy and pneumonia, just as she was starting a new job at a bank: "I remember feeling sick and I was worried: *Man, I can't be sick, I just got this job, they're going to fire me.* We'd only been married for two months and my husband was giving me a lot of grief. He told me, 'Your family warned me about you. They said you were over this, and we're supposed to have our whole lives ahead of us.' So of course I went to work. I walked into the bank and got like tunnel vision and heard echoing, and that's the last thing I remember."

When she woke up, she was in a hospital emergency room. She learned that her entire life had been turned upside down when she collapsed in the bank: "My coworkers called my husband and they also called 911. Apparently my husband got there first, and from what my coworkers later told me, he was really angry with me, because he said he didn't have time for this. Thankfully he dropped me off at the hospital. He told the doctor, 'I can't take care of her. I didn't sign up for this.' I never saw him again. After dropping me off at the hospital, he went home and he packed his bags and he applied for immediate deployment in Iraq. I don't know what was more shocking, that he disappeared or that I woke up in the hospital. (Three years later I got a phone call. He said, 'It's me. Are you still sick? Because I'd like to try and work on things.' I told him I was still sick, and he hung up the phone. And that was it.)"

In the emergency room Starr received a long overdue gift: an accurate diagnosis. The ER doctor told her that she had a condition called long QT syndrome, a heart rhythm disorder, as well as a dysfunctional mitral valve. (Some athletes who die suddenly on the field are felled by undiagnosed long QT syndrome.) When diagnosed in a timely matter, the condition can be treatable.[33] Starr's heart disease most likely would have been detected in childhood if someone had given her standard cardiac tests instead of dismissing her symptoms as a ploy to get attention.

When Starr collapsed at the bank, she experienced cardiac arrest. A cardiac surgeon saved her life and operated on her, inserting a device combining a pacemaker and an implantable cardioverter defibrillator (ICD), which uses electrical pulses and shocks to control life-threatening arrhythmias and to get the heart beating again. (Pacemakers are typically used when the heart beats too slowly. ICDs are advised for patients at risk for sudden cardiac death. Some patients, like Starr, have a device that combines both functions.)[34]

Rather than being bitter or angry, Starr initially was thrilled to finally have a diagnosis: "I can honestly tell you I felt like a new person, I was the happiest I'd been in my entire life, because I wasn't crazy—I was sick. Even now it gives me chills. *I told you guys I was sick!* It was clarity. . . . They didn't just misdiagnose me for so many years, they didn't diagnose me at all."

Because she went untreated until she was in her twenties, her heart was permanently damaged and there has been no easy fix. She's had more than two dozen surgeries and endured more than two hundred shocks from multiple ICD devices. When we talked in 2017, Starr was in her late thirties and was on her fourth ICD. Less than a year later, she was facing another operation to fix the ICD leads, the wires that connect the device to the heart. (A 2012 study concluded that "women who underwent ICD implantation had greater risks for complications and were less likely to experience appropriate ICD-delivered therapies than men."[35] Six years later, another study again found that complications with implanted ICDs were significantly more common in women. Researchers pointed out that many of the clinical trials of ICDs had small numbers of women.)[36]

One positive life change came out of her ordeal: When Starr's husband bolted, he didn't even bother to inform her family of her medical crisis. After not hearing from his granddaughter, Starr's worried grandfather got in his car and drove from South Carolina to Florida. Finding Starr's home empty, he drove to the bank where she worked, but no one could tell him where she was. Numerous phone calls later, it was discovered that Starr was still in the hospital; one of her coworkers, who was a medical school student, accompanied her grandfather to the hospital. This coworker ended up sticking around and helping Starr's family. "He was able to talk with the doctors and explain to my family what was going on, that's how we became friends," said Starr.

As she recovered, their friendship grew, until one day Starr asked him: "Are we dating?" They were. (When we first talked, they had been married for eight years.) "Sometimes I wake up in the morning and my husband is checking my pulse," said Starr.

In addition to her physical problems, Starr also believes she has post-traumatic stress from the years she was misdiagnosed: "I still have fear when I feel sick and when I go to a doctor of not being believed, of being treated like I'm crazy. It hinders me, which upsets my husband, because he's a physician. He says, 'Look, it's obvious you're sick.' And I tell him, 'You don't get it; there are doctors out there who treat women like it's all in their heads.'"

Too sick to work, Starr became a volunteer for WomenHeart, as well as a speaker and advocate for the women's organization Hadassah, which in 2016 launched the Coalition for Women's Health Equity.[37] In a moving talk in 2018 for hundreds of delegates at a Hadassah Women's Health Empowerment Summit in Washington, DC, Starr talked about turning her negative medical experiences into something positive. She has discovered that her story resonates with other women who struggle with an "invisible" or misdiagnosed disease. In her speech, Starr reflected that if even one person "had just listened to me and believed that I was sick, that one person would have changed my entire world. The physical and mental suffering I have endured and the lifelong damage it caused would have been considerably less. My hope is that I bring comfort and solace to other women like myself, regardless of age, race, ethnicity, who may be struggling at any stage of heart disease or illness. Listen to your body.

You know your body better than anybody. You are not a faker. You are not dramatic. And you are not alone. If my story can impact one person and result in a better outcome for them, then I have truly achieved. Today, I strive to be a person I needed when I was younger."[38]

"NO ONE BELIEVED THAT I WAS SERIOUSLY SICK"

A 2016 scientific statement by the AHA noted that while all female heart attack patients face worse outcomes than do men, the risk factors for Black and Hispanic women are even more pronounced. Dr. Mehta, who served as chair of the writing group, said in a press release that despite improvements in cardiovascular deaths over the last decade, women (especially women of color) still fare worse than men, with their heart disease underdiagnosed and undertreated.[39]

Cecilia (not her real name), who is Latina, has always been thin, healthy, and very active, enjoying hiking, dancing, and Jazzercise. In 2016, when she was fifty-five, she was working as a hospital stress management specialist while also studying in graduate school. Out of the blue, she began to experience overwhelming fatigue.

"I was noticing that it was getting more and more difficult for me to just even walk around the block," she said. "Right before the Christmas holidays, I wasn't having any pain, I just felt very, very tired and I was having trouble moving around. My son came home for Christmas break and he said, 'Mom, you're not even getting halfway down the block.' I told him, 'Yeah, I just feel so tired, I feel like I'm going to drop.'"

When she started to have some chest pain and nausea, she went to urgent care, where she was diagnosed with walking pneumonia and asthma. No tests were performed, and she was sent home with an inhaler, which did nothing to improve her symptoms, so Cecilia followed up with her primary care doctor. He thought the problems were respiratory in nature, but just to be sure, he gave her a referral to a cardiologist; that doctor couldn't see her for six weeks. Meanwhile, Cecilia went to a respiratory specialist who did several tests. "Even walking down the hall with the special testing devices, I couldn't breathe. I thought I was going to pass out," she said.

But all of the breathing tests came back normal and there was no urgency on the specialist's part to investigate further. Cecilia's husband implored the doctor to do something: "You can see that she can't walk and she can't breathe. This is so completely the opposite of my wife. She's a very active person."

When Cecilia finally saw a cardiologist, she asked to have a stress test, but he did not think this was necessary. Feeling desperate and disillusioned, Cecilia had a consult with another doctor at the hospital where she worked, a female integrative medicine specialist who also was a cardiologist. After listening to her description of her symptoms and doing a clinical exam, this doctor immediately referred Cecilia to a heart surgeon, who performed a coronary angiogram, an X-ray used to look at blood vessels in the heart.

Shortly after the procedure began, Cecilia became aware that something was not right. She was put under and rushed to the operating room. "When I woke up, the doctor said, 'I had to go in and save your life. You had a 98 percent blockage on your left descending artery. If I had waited a day, you would have died.' So I went from a diagnosis of 'asthma and walking pneumonia' to 'almost died,'" said Cecilia. "After my care, I did go into some depression because I was in shock. I couldn't believe that somebody healthy like me, that this could happen. I never looked ill. No one believed I was seriously sick."

Cecilia felt that she was released much too quickly from the hospital—on the same day that the stent was put in. Then she had to fight to get a referral for cardiac rehab. (After a heart attack or heart surgery, women are less likely than men to be referred for cardiac rehab, considered by experts to be an essential component of recovery.)[40]

Dr. Minissian of the Smidt Heart Institute described cardiac rehab as "imperative. Exercise plays such a huge role in our vascular health. Implementing early exercise is important. Back in the day, when I was a nurse twenty-plus years ago, we used to put people in bed and let them rest there. Now we have people out of bed within hours after their surgery. We know that getting them up and getting them going is really important. Cardiac rehab is a regulated, supervised program that gives very distinct doses of exercise under the supervision of an exercise physiologist or a registered nurse. It gets people back up and going with their fitness."

Dr. Minissian continued: "This really helps for blood vessel health. When we exercise we excrete our own nitric oxide, which helps to dilate our blood vessels. The lining of the blood vessels is called the endothelium. It's kind of like your skin. For a lot of people who've had surgery or they've had stents put in, that endothelium can be injured. The exercise helps to reduce inflammation and to make sure that the endothelium can get back to being healthy again."

When Cecilia pushed to get into cardiac rehab, she was told that she didn't look sick and could recover on her own. Still, she persisted in asking for a referral, and eventually got one—but her time in cardiac rehab turned out to be a negative experience: "I finally went to cardiac rehab and it was predominantly men—and I was hit on! I'm thinking, *Seriously? I'm here to get better.* It was uncomfortable, to say the least." (A 2016 Canadian study found that female cardiac patients had improvements in anxiety, depression, and diet when they attended women-only cardiac rehab sessions.)[41]

Cecilia described her post-care experience as "daunting, because they expected me to bounce back. . . . I was in and out of the hospital. Shortly after, I became nauseous and had some follow-up issues from scarring with the stents. . . . I didn't know what any of it meant. I woke up and I'm being told, 'We just saved your life.' Are you kidding me? What are you talking about? My family was in shock. It was a challenge for my husband because he had never seen me sick, so that was hard. My son saw me fall one time in the midst of the post-care because I just wasn't feeling well."

Well-wishers always seemed to have a story to tell Cecilia about someone else with heart disease who had recovered in a matter of weeks. These stories made her feel worse, especially when she was still not herself months after having the stents put in: "None of the doctors to this day has honored or explained to me why I was still so tired. They kind of made me feel like it was all in my head. . . . I was still working—it's not like I wasn't doing anything—but I would come home feeling absolutely wiped out, like I had gone on a marathon. Nobody warned me."

It wasn't until she joined WomenHeart and heard other women's stories that Cecilia learned that there is no universal timetable for recovery. Some people feel better in a few weeks, but for others the process can take much longer.

"In my post-care, I was fatigued for almost an entire year. People asked, 'What's the problem? What aren't you okay?' I'm an incredibly positive person and I was trying, but I just couldn't do it. My chest hurt, I didn't feel good, I was nauseous, so that was disconcerting for me. There was a lack of compassion and empathy in the aftercare. The whole experience was a shock to me," she said.

Cecilia had no idea what caused her heart disease, especially since she has always been thin and active. She wondered if one factor might be the preeclampsia she experienced during one of her pregnancies. (Preeclampsia is a pregnancy complication that can come on suddenly and may be life-threatening to both the mother and baby. It is characterized by high blood pressure and potential damage to the liver and kidneys.)[42] After her pregnancy, no one talked to Cecilia about future cardiac problems or discussed monitoring her heart health.

"I recently learned that women who have this, years later, there can be issues with heart disease. I discovered that on my own. Even when I mentioned it to my current cardiologist, he just said, 'Well, that might be,'" Cecilia said.

A study published in 2017 found that preeclampsia is associated with an increased risk of death from cardiovascular disease. The researchers concluded that this "highlights the importance of lifelong monitoring of cardiovascular risk factors in women with a history of preeclampsia."[43]

When we last spoke, Cecilia was feeling better and was back to her active lifestyle. She was thankful for the cardiologist who correctly diagnosed her and for the surgeon who saved her life. To the doctors who misdiagnosed her for six months she had this to say: "Stop dismissing women; stop dismissing us, as if this is all some Victorian era 'female' malady. There's something real going on. We're trying to convey it to the best of our abilities. Sometimes we have the words; sometimes we don't. Please, please, please believe us."

5

CHRONIC

Autoimmune diseases, chronic fatigue syndrome, and fibromyalgia are distinct afflictions, but they tend to share a common symptom—acute disbelief. Many women who are stricken with these debilitating conditions become shell-shocked after being catapulted from good health to sudden and severe illness. And the doctors they turn to for help sometimes refuse to accept that something is physically wrong with their desperate patients. The long-ingrained skepticism about women's symptoms is due in part to how little of medical school education focuses on chronic illnesses that more often strike women. In a *New Yorker* review of books about long-term ailments, writer Lidija Haas noted that "there's a class of illnesses—multi-symptomatic, chronic, hard to diagnose—that remain associated with suffering women and disbelieving experts. . . . [I]t isn't only a question of whether or not individual patients are believed. An enigmatic disorder that might have justified a great influx of research money and ingenuity has instead remained stalled and under-investigated, with key players unable to agree on basic facts, such as what it does, how to tell who has it, and what, if anything, can treat it."[1]

FRIENDLY FIRE

It's not known why autoimmune diseases are on the rise, but researchers suspect that possible causes are infections, viruses, and genetics, as well as physical and emotional trauma. It's thought that our widespread exposure to thousands of environmental toxins used in industry, commerce, and agriculture may play a role.[2] A 2016 study found a link between increases in certain autoimmune diseases and additives in processed foods.[3] Societal and personal upheaval also may contribute. Researchers at the University of Iceland in Reykjavik found that people who had experienced intense stress and trauma had a 36 percent increased risk of developing forty-one autoimmune diseases.[4]

While each autoimmune disease—which can range from mild to life-threatening—has different symptoms, a common factor is that the body mistakenly attacks itself, a process compared to friendly fire. The inflammation caused by autoimmune diseases can damage organs, skin, tissues, joints, muscles, and blood cells. Some 50 million Americans have an autoimmune disease, and, for reasons that remain largely a mystery, about 75 percent are women.[5] According to the nonprofit advocacy group the American Autoimmune Related Diseases Association (AARDA), autoimmune disease is one of the ten leading causes of death in female children and women in all age groups up to sixty-four years old.[6] Delayed diagnosis is common and can worsen symptoms and prognosis; on average patients see four doctors over a period of three years before finding out what is wrong.

"In autoimmune diseases, the patient has to be proactive. There is no 'autoimmunologist,' and that's a problem," AARDA president and executive director Virginia T. Ladd said, adding that patients often go from specialist to specialist in search of answers.

Most patients share one early hallmark symptom—extreme fatigue. "That symptom is dismissed by doctors 85 percent of the time," said Ms. Ladd. (In fact, she recommended that women never tell a doctor they are tired but instead say that they are "functionally exhausted"—a phrase that sometimes yields more respect in a medical setting.) Researchers have identified eighty to one hundred autoimmune diseases, and experts believe there most likely are others not yet named. Ms. Ladd said, "Each disease is relatively rare, but looking at them collectively, that's another story."

Internist Dr. Abid Khan, director of the Autoimmune Center at Mid-Michigan Health, told *SELF* magazine that he started an autoimmune disease clinic after his wife nearly died from undiagnosed lupus.[7] In Pittsburgh, Allegheny Health Network opened the Autoimmunity Institute in 2018, under the direction of rheumatologist Dr. Susan M. Manzi, who also serves as medical director for the nonprofit advocacy group Lupus Foundation of America. Dr. Manzi described the institute as a game changer for autoimmune patients, with more than twenty-five clinicians representing twelve subspecialties "all working under one roof in the same space and managing all the different organ systems that can be impacted in autoimmune diseases. The institute also offers access to cutting-edge research and to clinical trials testing new treatments."

In Blackfoot, Idaho, Dr. David Bilstrom—who is certified in physical medicine and rehabilitation, functional, and regenerative medicine and acupuncture—leads the Bingham Memorial Center for Functional Medicine and International Autoimmune Institute, which was launched in 2015. "We tend to see people who have been everywhere, going to lots of doctors before they end up here. By the time they get to us they have so many organ systems involved, all at the same time," said Dr. Bilstrom.

Once a woman develops one autoimmune condition, she's more vulnerable to other assaults on her health. The most common autoimmune diseases in women are rheumatoid arthritis, type 1 diabetes, lupus, autoimmune thyroid disease, inflammatory bowel disease, Sjogren's syndrome, and multiple sclerosis. (Lyme disease sometimes is misdiagnosed as an autoimmune disorder, but it is a bacterial tick-borne infection that must be treated with antibiotics. Left untreated, Lyme disease can cause long-term health problems. As with so many other ailments, men and women present differently with Lyme disease, and women often have a tougher time getting diagnosed.)[8]

When I interviewed her for the *Los Angeles Times*, Ms. Ladd said that the main concern of women with autoimmune diseases is that doctors don't hear what they are saying: "Indeed, some 40 percent of women who eventually are found to have a serious autoimmune disease have been told by a physician that they are complainers or simply too concerned with their health. When these women finally find out what's wrong, they are thankful, even if they know for certain that they have a chronic condition."[9]

Sometimes, the first step toward a diagnosis is made when a primary care physician suspects an autoimmune disease and orders lab work to check if there are antinuclear antibodies (ANA) in a patient's blood. One issue is that these tests are not foolproof; sick individuals can have normal results and healthy people may have positive ANA tests. In most cases, though, a positive ANA test will get the patient referred to a rheumatologist for more specific testing.

Patients may end up going to several rheumatologists before getting answers, especially with the less common autoimmune disorders. "The disease that I specialize in, scleroderma, is quite rare, so most of the time patients who come to me have already seen five or six doctors. Sometimes they have been diagnosed correctly, other times not," explained Dr. Elizabeth R. Volkmann, a UCLA rheumatologist whose research focuses on the gastrointestinal, vascular, and pulmonary aspects of scleroderma (also called systemic sclerosis) a sometimes life-threatening rheumatologic disease, affecting more women than men, in which the skin and internal organs are attacked.

Depending on the diagnosis, rheumatologists typically consult with other specialists for help in managing symptoms. For example, patients with chronic inflammatory bowel conditions, such as Crohn's disease or ulcerative colitis, need to be cared for by a gastroenterologist experienced in treating autoimmune diseases that affect the digestive tract. Patients with lupus, a life-threatening systemic disease that can harm every part of the body, may need to see multiple specialists, including cardiologists, dermatologists, and nephrologists. "We always say, it takes a team to manage lupus patients," said Dr. Manzi.

"I'M HERE BECAUSE I NEED HELP"

Growing up in Texas, Wendy Rodgers was healthy and athletic, playing basketball and volleyball and running track. She had a daughter when she was sixteen, by unmedicated childbirth, with no complications. When Wendy was twenty-five she married a man from California, and the family moved to Los Angeles. Not long after, she developed uncomfortable joint pain. "I thought that once I acclimated to the weather in Southern California, I'd be okay, but as time went on it didn't get better; it got worse. I would wake up feeling achy. My mobility was decreasing. I felt like an old lady," said Wendy.

One morning she found she could barely move. "It was like I was paralyzed, I couldn't even lift my head up from the pillow. That scared me so bad. And I realized that this is not normal for a twenty-seven-year-old. I knew something was really wrong."

Wendy went to her primary care physician, wanting to discuss her joint pain and mobility problems. But the appointment never got beyond checking her vital signs, because her blood pressure was 225 over 125, well above normal. Wendy had never before had high blood pressure, yet no one thought to question why it now was skyrocketing. "Because I'm an African American woman and I'm not the skinniest woman, it was just basically assumed that I wasn't eating right and that I wasn't taking care of myself. That was the profile I was given, without any further investigation as to why my blood pressure would have suddenly been that high," she said.

Classified as a hypertension patient, Wendy was put on a series of different blood pressure medications, none of which worked. Meanwhile, her joint pain grew worse, her hair started to fall out in clumps, and she developed rashes. Wendy—a middle school science teacher who then had a bachelor's degree in biology and later earned two master's degrees, in education and public health—started to conduct her own research. In a book about women's health issues, she found a chapter with a short description of systemic lupus erythematosus, an autoimmune disease that can cause inflammation throughout the body, damaging joints, kidneys, the brain, heart, and lungs. Early symptoms may include fatigue, joint pain, and rashes.[10] Wendy was struck by how much it sounded like what she was experiencing. Armed with this new information, she went back to her primary care doctor: "I asked him if lupus could be a possibility, because I saw it was something that was common in women, especially African American women, and it often caused joint pain. It was like a light bulb moment for him. He told me, 'I hadn't even thought of that.' The doctor and I were both kind of excited over the realization that 'this could be it.'"

She was referred to a rheumatologist, who did not share her excitement about possibly having solved the mystery of her failing health. The first question he asked Wendy was why she was there. "Now, I'm sure he knew why I was there, because I had to be referred," Wendy pointed out. "He was very dismissive and really rude. He had these beautiful blue eyes. I remember looking at his eyes when I listened to him, and I realized that this man didn't understand that I was suffering."

Wendy was taken aback when the rheumatologist theorized that it's not uncommon for people to see an illness described in a TV commercial and to think that they have it. She tried to describe her symptoms, her research, and her suspicion that she might have lupus. This seemed to annoy the doctor, who clearly resented that she did her own investigation of her illness. Confronted with his attitude, Wendy became angry, but she made a conscious decision to hide her emotions and to try a different tactic: "So I put myself in a very humble place. I told him, 'I understand that you're the doctor. I'm here because I need help, and I don't have the tools to help myself.'"

Wendy's instincts were correct—her deliberate words soothed the doctor's ego and got the appointment on track; the rheumatologist announced that he was going to order some lab work. He added that he would throw in a blood test for lupus, almost as an afterthought, "as if he were doing me a favor," Wendy recalled.

A few days later Wendy received a call telling her to return to the rheumatologist. His arrogance and lack of compassion now were gone, replaced with solemnity as he informed Wendy that she did, indeed, have lupus. She took the news calmly, which surprised the doctor, who told her that most patients cry when they get the diagnosis. At that point Wendy was relieved to finally have an answer for what was wrong. She left the doctor's office with a name for her condition—but little else. She was not given any instructions on ways to manage her symptoms or how to avoid disease flare-ups. She had no idea of the challenges ahead.

"I didn't really understand the impact it could have on my heath. He didn't tell me how dangerous it is and how devastating it could be on your life," she recalled.

Unaware that heat and sunlight could trigger lupus flare-ups, Wendy went with friends for a weekend in Palm Springs, where she spent hours in the sun. When she was back in Los Angeles, she consulted with a dermatologist for help with the terrible rashes that now plagued her. When he told her she needed to be diligent about avoiding the sun, she was stunned and said she had just been in the desert. "That doctor looked at me and he said, 'Wendy, you need to take this seriously.' I said, 'I am, I just didn't know.' He said, 'You could have a massive heart attack and die. You could have kidney failure and die.' He told me about other dire complications, and they all ended in 'and die.'"

One of her lab tests showed a problem with her kidneys, so she was referred to a nephrologist, but there were no appointments for the next three months. As she waited to see the specialist, she took a turn for the worse. Her mother urged her to try to be seen sooner. Wendy called a few times but still couldn't get an immediate appointment. After a while, she gave up. "I can't even really describe how weak I felt. I didn't have the energy mentally and physically to advocate for myself; I wasn't in that place, that's how drained I was. I had never felt like that in my life, I was out of it. I would get dressed and lay on the couch," Wendy remembered.

By the time she had the appointment, her body was swollen, her shoes no longer fit, and her skin was so tight it was painful to the touch. Wendy did not know that these were signs of kidney failure. The alarmed nephrologist told her she needed to have a kidney biopsy to determine the best treatment course. What should have been a simple procedure turned into nineteen days in the hospital because her blood pressure was still raging out of control. Wendy learned that some medications react differently in African Americans.[11] "That was the case with me, so what was happening was that a lot of the things that are the standard of care didn't work. That was a lot of the frustration and hardship with my case; it just wasn't like you could go to a textbook and find a solution. With lupus, it doesn't have a pattern; it's unpredictable, and the severity can be different in people. You have to figure it out, because there are all these pathways in the body that can be affected. It's a very complex disease," she said.

When she finally was able to have the biopsy, the test revealed severe kidney damage. Wendy ended up in the ICU for six months, where she faced multiple complications: "I had four grand mal seizures, I lost the ability to walk, I ended up losing all of my hair doing chemotherapy, I developed two rare blood disorders, and I had fluid on my brain. I was hanging on to life by a thread; it was a horrible fight."

As her ongoing health crisis destroyed her marriage and derailed her teaching career, she learned firsthand how stress can aggravate lupus symptoms. Wendy credits her hematologist at Kaiser Permanente in Los Angeles with making unique efforts to save her life, especially when other doctors were skeptical that she could have developed two rare blood disorders at the same time. "He searched and searched for a specialist and he finally found a doctor in Canada who told him how to treat me."

Wendy, who described herself as a devout Christian, praised the hematologist for the years of care he gave her: "My hematologist ended up being like a father to me. That was the doctor whom I trusted the most. He is a Jewish man, a gentle, caring soul."

Wendy was on dialysis for nine years. During that time she couldn't work as a teacher, so she started volunteering as an advocate for the

Lupus Foundation of America and, later, for two other organizations: OneLegacy, dedicated to saving lives through organ transplants, and the Renal Support Network, which helps patients living with kidney disease. In 2009 Wendy received a new kidney from an anonymous donor. The surgery went well, but because transplant patients must take immunosuppressants to prevent organ rejection, they are at constant risk for infections. Wendy understandably was worried about returning to work in the classroom, since teachers are exposed to so many student illnesses. But the kidney doctor in charge of her post-transplant care dismissed Wendy's concerns and refused to help her get the work modifications she needed. "He not only disregarded my fear but he incorrectly assumed that I didn't want to work." In fact, Wendy very much wanted to continue working, but without the risks posed by being in a classroom. She tried without success to explain to the kidney doctor that she needed time to recover and to earn a second master's degree, which would allow her to embark on a new career path—one that would not put her health in jeopardy.

Wendy ended up returning to the classroom, teaching science to middle school students in a private Christian school in Koreatown in Los Angeles: "I'm the only African American teacher there. This is my first time being immersed in the Asian community. I love it! I teach my kids about lupus. We even do a lupus awareness day. I've been very open about how it's affected my health. Who knows? One of these kids may end up becoming a doctor. I tell my students, 'If you're going to become a doctor, you need to know this.'"

Despite her harrowing medical journey, Wendy said that she considers herself fortunate because it did not take her years to get an accurate diagnosis. (She was too modest to say that her diagnosis was expedited largely through her own efforts at researching her symptoms and bringing her findings to the attention of her doctors.)

The process of getting a diagnosis can be particularly challenging for Black and Latina women. Linda Goler Blount, president and CEO of the nonprofit advocacy organization the Black Women's Health Imperative, said that when women of color try to discuss autoimmune symptoms in a doctor's office "physicians are less likely to even think about lupus. They're more likely to come to other conclusions, based on their interpretation of lifestyle and what women are doing. Rather than come to a conclusion earlier that maybe this is an autoimmune disorder, they're more interested in telling women, 'Well, you need to stop smoking or drinking' or 'You need to lose weight.' It becomes a problem for the woman to solve herself. The message is that she's at fault—but of course we know that's not the case for autoimmune disorders."

Black women tend to develop lupus at a younger age, during their childbearing years, and they suffer more serious complications. A large study done by researchers at Emory University confirmed that the disease disproportionately affects Black women. Principal investigator Dr. S. Sam Lim said in a news release about the study: "These are young women in the prime of their careers, family and fertility. This means a severely compromised future with a disease that waxes and wanes, affecting every aspect of daily living for the rest of their lives." [12]

Dr. Manzi said that one cause of misdiagnosis of lupus is a lack of awareness of the illness among doctors, due in part to how little time is devoted in medical schools and training programs to studying autoimmune disease. In addition, lupus is particularly challenging to recognize. "Lupus patients are like snowflakes; no two are alike. They can present with a wide spectrum of problems that can range from mild to severe, but they can look different in everyone," said Dr. Manzi, explaining that lupus can affect any and all organ systems in the body.

Doctors need to pay attention to "who is walking in the door," said Dr. Manzi, especially if that patient is a young woman with classic lupus symptoms like fevers, fatigue, rashes, and joint pain, "because 90 percent of people with lupus are women, and the vast majority are between the ages of fifteen and forty-five, and there's about a threefold increased risk in African American women, Hispanic women, and Asian American women. Your antenna should go up for patients in those ethnic groups." (Native American women also are at increased risk for lupus.)

Even though 1.5 million people in the United States have lupus, only 72 percent of Americans between the ages of eighteen and thirty-four—the population most likely to get the disease—know anything at all about it, according to the Lupus Foundation of America. [13]

"There's not only lack of awareness among people themselves who can be impacted by the disease, but also physicians," said Dr. Manzi. "When you're training to be a physician, you learn an awful lot about heart disease and cancer. But exposure to information about autoimmune diseases is underrepresented."

A lot of women with autoimmune diseases end up coping on their own, without support or understanding. Dr. Manzi told me about one of her patients, a young woman who lives in a close-knit neighborhood where the moms hang out together. When one of the mothers was stricken with breast cancer, the neighborhood group rallied to help her with child-care and meals. At the same time, Dr. Manzi's patient became seriously ill with lupus and had to have chemotherapy. "No one did anything," said Dr. Manzi. "Her friends understood breast cancer, but they didn't under-stand lupus. That same lack of compassion and empathy that you can often see when someone is diagnosed with lupus is a reflection of the general lack of awareness and understanding of the disease. . . . [I]t is a condition that has slipped through the cracks."

"SICK AND TIRED OF BEING SICK AND TIRED"

Even a supposedly mild autoimmune disease can be life-altering. Like many women, Clara (not her real name) is a busy lady. She works four days a week while also managing her elderly mother's care and babysit-ting for her young grandchildren. There are times when she does all this while not feeling very well.

Clara's mysterious symptoms started in 1995, when she was in her early forties. At the time, in addition to working full-time, she also volun-teered in her daughters' elementary school. One day she "started feeling ill, with these vague symptoms that were annoying and persistent, such as low-grade fevers, headachy, intermittent sore throat, first you're sweating and then you're feeling cold, things like that. I didn't really know what was wrong with me. It went on for a long time."

Her primary care doctor diagnosed a viral infection and said that it would go away soon. But Clara's symptoms worsened, with the onset of severe pain in the joints of her wrists, hips, and knees. "Not only was my doctor not really paying attention to me, other than shrugging his shoul-ders and saying, 'Take Tylenol,' he didn't conduct any lab tests either."

This went on for months. A coworker who saw how sick Clara was urged her to get a second opinion and recommended a doctor. Clara made an appointment, not realizing that this physician actually was a respirato-ry specialist (and Clara was not having any breathing problems). Nevertheless, Clara was impressed by the doctor's caring attitude and listening skills.

The physician took particular note of Clara's volunteer work in her daughters' school. Numerous blood tests were ordered. "She made me feel a little hopeful because she didn't look at me like I was crazy," said Clara. "At that point, I was sick and tired of being sick and tired. I wanted some answers."

The blood tests revealed that Clara had contracted a parvovirus, most likely from close contact with students carrying fifth disease, a common and highly contagious childhood ailment characterized by bright red cheeks and a rash. With adults, the main symptom is joint pain lasting for days or weeks.[14]

In Clara's case, the joint pain never went away. Because one of her blood tests revealed an elevated rheumatoid factor, she was referred to a rheumatologist, who ordered still more lab tests. But Clara didn't test positive for anything, and her doctors were at a loss to explain what was wrong. After conducting her own research, Clara now believes she has a "tweak" in her immune system, most likely triggered by the parvovirus. "What it did, like any kind of virus or infection can do, it caused my immune system to go a little haywire. It was some kind of challenge to my body," she speculated. "Before that time, I never had a single health problem. I always bounced back from everything. But this was something else and it was never-ending."

She still gets occasional attacks and has had multiple surgeries to repair her knees, which, she thinks, were permanently damaged by the decades-long assault of the mystery illness on her joints. She suspects that infections, stress, and fatigue are triggers for flare-ups. Clara remains grateful to the respiratory doctor she saw more than twenty years ago, who first took her symptoms seriously: "She was listening and putting the pieces together. She was a good doctor."

Often, women have no idea what causes their symptoms. One of my cousins, Riya Zelcer, was on her feet for more than three decades in her job as a hospital neonatal nurse. In 2009 she suddenly began to experience severe leg cramps, although that description minimizes the agony she felt each time an attack happened. She described the episodes as "horrible spasms in my leg, where my toes and foot got pulled back so hard, so violently, that it literally felt like my toes were going to break off. It was very painful, and it was happening up to ten times a day, so I was just really panicking. . . . I went to a few doctors who couldn't figure out what it was."

Eventually, a neurologist sent Riya for a brain MRI. The imaging test was done without contrast dye and showed nothing irregular. (When Riya told me this, I was puzzled—I've had dozens of MRIs over the years and they are always done using contrast dye. The dye functions as a highlighter, illuminating subtle abnormalities.) Riya said she didn't know why the doctor ordered the scan without dye. At the time, however, she was thankful that the test didn't reveal anything irregular.

With no answers about the cause of the debilitating spasms, they suddenly went away. Riya was, of course, relieved and returned to her normal life of working as a neonatal nurse. She assumed that whatever her mysterious ailment was, it must have disappeared. But that was not the case.

"Four years ago, all of a sudden in the middle of the night, I had a dream. You know how when you go under water and you're just about at the surface to take a big gulp of air and then somebody pulls you down? My brothers used to do that to me and it scared me. So I had that dream, that I was just at the surface and then somebody pulled me down," she said. "And then I woke up with one of those horrible spasms. That was the first time in four years that I'd had one."

She went to see another neurologist, who ordered an MRI, this time with contrast dye. The test showed that Riya has multiple sclerosis (MS), a disease in which the immune system attacks myelin, the protective sheaths of nerve cells in the brain and spinal cord, causing problems in the central nervous system. Riya now is on medication and uses a cane to help her walk. I asked if she thought her delayed diagnosis might have altered the course of the disease—or, to put it another way: If she had started the medication earlier, would her prognosis be better today? "I'm not 100 percent sure," Riya said, adding that the medication now seems to be keeping her symptoms at bay.

Riya pointed out that her symptoms are not typical of MS, and that when she got the leg cramps in her forties, she was older than most women diagnosed with the disease. But she also believes her original doctors did not dig deep enough. "When they couldn't figure out the diagnosis the first time, they were just kind of throwing their hands up in the air. One of the doctors wanted me to show him a cramp. I was so terrified of the cramps, I didn't want to try to have one. I did actually have an attack in the office, but he didn't witness it. I described it and he just said he didn't know what it was."

I first experienced vague autoimmune and neurological symptoms back in 2000. My doctors concluded that I had Guillain-Barré syndrome, a disorder in which the immune system attacks the nervous system, causing numbness and sometimes paralysis. There are tests used to diagnose Guillain-Barré syndrome, but my doctors did not order those. They simply said I eventually would recover.

After finally being correctly diagnosed with a nonmalignant brain tumor via an MRI scan with contrast dye in 2005, I was fortunate to end up in the gifted hands of esteemed neurosurgeon Dr. Keith Black at Cedars-Sinai Medical Center in Los Angeles. During my first consult with Dr. Black, I asked him about the Guillain-Barré diagnosis that I mistakenly had been given. Dr. Black explained that any brain tumor—especially one that sits inside your skull for years—can scramble your autoimmune system, sending incorrect signals throughout the body and producing multiple symptoms that can mimic other diseases. The mistake my previous doctors had made was failing to investigate why my autoimmune symptoms persisted.

I thought my successful brain surgery would end my autoimmune issues, but I was wrong. A few years after my craniotomy, I suddenly began to get severe pains in both hands. My primary care physician ordered blood tests, one of which revealed an elevated rheumatoid factor. I was referred to a highly regarded rheumatologist at West Hills Hospital in the San Fernando Valley. The doctor walked into the exam room and, without even looking at me or introducing himself, asked: "So, what's your story of woe?"

We could dismiss that question by saying the doctor had terrible bedside manner. But I suspected his comment revealed a jaded view of the many female patients who came to him for help. It was a condescending assessment of their serious problems as mere "stories of woe" that seemed to be taking up his valuable time. Do I even need to say that I didn't stay with this doctor? (And I later learned from another rheumatologist, who was kind and caring, that I don't have rheumatoid arthritis.)

FIBROMYALGIA AND CHRONIC FATIGUE SYNDROME

By the time Sue Ingebretson, author of the book *FibroWHYalgia* was in her thirties, she had been to dozens of doctors. Her confusing ailments started as a teenager, when she was plagued by digestive issues, trouble swallowing, and joint pain, as well as problems with walking and balance. When she was in her twenties, she suddenly developed severe chest pain and saw a cardiologist. He took one look at her and declared: "Come back when you're a man, when you smoke three packs a day, and when you're over three hundred pounds." (She later learned that the chest pain and trouble breathing were not heart related but were due to costochondritis, an inflammation of the cartilage that connects the ribs to the breastbone.) At one point she had more than two dozen strange symptoms, and no one could tell her why she felt so lousy, especially when most of her lab tests were normal. Finally, when she was thirty-nine, a doctor she had consulted with multiple times called her, excited to announce that he finally had solved the mystery of her bad health: "He told me that he had figured out the answer. . . . He said he realized that what was going on was that I was afraid of getting older. I was so shocked I didn't know what to say or how to answer. He told me: 'You're an attractive woman and you're aging, that must be frightening.' I never saw him again."

She started doing her own research in college libraries, reading about conditions that sounded a lot like her own. A breakthrough came after she created a spreadsheet linking her symptoms with what was going on in her life at the time. In the process of documenting some of her most symptomatic days, she realized that she often felt worse after a medical or dental procedure, while taking birth control pills, or after a particularly stressful or exhausting event. Armed with this information, Sue took her spreadsheet to a new general practitioner. "I think I have fibromyalgia," Sue told her. After looking over all of the paperwork that Sue had provided, as well as her medical records, the doctor surprised her by declaring: "No duh." Almost twenty years later, Sue still remembers how she felt when the physician said those words: "It was like walking into the Land of Oz in color." The doctor also stressed to Sue that the journey to feeling better would be guided by "10 percent doctor and 90 percent patient."

Sue eventually came to believe that she had been made vulnerable to getting a chronic health condition because of the circumstances of her impoverished childhood, where the staples of her diet were processed cheese and crackers. "I grew up with absolutely no understanding of, or experience with, healthy nutrition at all. We ate poorly . . . not a vegetable in sight."

When she was in high school, in 1976, the government launched a national swine flu immunization program, fearing that the world was about to be hit with a global epidemic. Sue ended up being given the vaccine three separate times at school because each of her extracurricular activities required students to be immunized. When she tried to explain that she had already been given the shot twice in the space of a few weeks, a nurse told her, "Oh, it's harmless" before injecting her a third time. As a teenager, Sue (who is five feet tall) weighed only seventy-eight pounds; she believes the triple dose of the vaccine was too much for her small body and wreaked havoc with her immune system.

Not long after getting the multiple shots, Sue was injured in a serious school bus accident. She now is certain that this event sealed the deal for her being stricken with fibromyalgia: "You pair together nutritional deficiency, the huge toxic exposure of heavy metals from the three doses of the swine flu vaccine, and then a serious accident—and you've got a recipe for the body being in trauma."

There is disagreement among experts about how to categorize fibromyalgia. Because it does not involve inflammation, it is not considered an autoimmune disease and is instead classified as a chronic nerve disorder. However you label it, the illness can cause unrelenting pain throughout the body. Extreme fatigue, depression, and insomnia also are common symptoms. The condition affects some 5 million Americans, 90 percent of them women. On average, it can take up to five years to get a diagnosis. Researchers who surveyed 670 fibromyalgia patients noted that patients experience "discouragement, rejection, suspicion, and stigma during their encounters with health care professionals," and that these encounters have a negative impact on their quality of life and symptoms. [15]

Treating fibromyalgia is challenging. As pointed out by *Consumer Reports*, the medications used to treat the illness include antidepressants, antiseizure drugs, and a muscle relaxant, but there is no clear evidence that these actually help patients. [16]

For years, fibromyalgia seemed to be considered a faux illness by much of the medical establishment, as if millions of women were somehow conjuring up the symptoms. A cynic might conclude that fibromyalgia only got the stamp of legitimacy when pharmaceutical companies did the math and concluded that there was big money to be made on women who were desperate for an effective treatment. Patients felt validated when Lyrica (pregabalin) and several other medications were given FDA approval—but many were disappointed after trying the drugs, which often didn't help and could have bad side effects. As I reported in the *Los Angeles Times*, a regular exercise program may be a more effective treatment than fibromyalgia meds for some patients.[17]

One consequence of the legitimization of fibromyalgia is that the ailment sometimes is a default diagnosis when women present with chronic pain. Dr. Sami Saba, a neurologist at Lenox Hill Hospital in New York City, explained that this can result in other painful conditions being missed. He told me about one of his patients who had severe skin pain. "She had been to several physicians, neurologists included. They did a bunch of tests, and they told her that they couldn't find anything, so her pain must be from fibromyalgia," said Dr. Saba. "Most patients with fibromyalgia have muscular pain through palpation of the muscles. Her pain was very different—it was burning, it felt hot, it was sensitive to just light touch and not to pressure on the muscle. When I examined her, it was in strange, patchy distribution, which also is atypical for fibromyalgia. I told her, 'You don't meet the criteria for fibromyalgia. You have unexplained pain syndrome and those are not the same.'"

Dr. Saba ordered a skin biopsy, which determined that the patient had a condition called small fiber neuropathy. "She started treatment with medications for neuropathic pain and she improved," said Dr. Saba. "She wasn't cured, but she did do much better after she was appropriately treated."

Bingham Memorial Center's Dr. Bilstrom said that patients with fibromyalgia and other painful conditions often face skepticism in medical settings: "Doctors order blood work and an X-ray and nothing shows up, so they conclude that the pain you're complaining about must be in your head. . . . [U]nfortunately, a lot of people are still told this."

Arlene Strategos, who has fibromyalgia, told me how grateful she is to have found a rheumatologist who really cares. She has stayed with him for more than two decades because "he was the first person who didn't discount it; he believed everything that I said. He has always treated me with respect."

When she was in her thirties and started to get pains in her head, neck, and arms, she suspected it was due to the repetitive motion strain that can occur with being a dental hygienist. But when she consulted different doctors, she was told her symptoms were due to the stress of being a single mother and "not to worry about it. . . . Then one day I was working on a patient and I couldn't move the thumb on my right hand."

A neurosurgeon told Arlene she had a problem with the discs in her neck, but that he didn't want to discuss surgery until she had tried every other possible treatment. "I tried every modality available, none of which helped. The pain I suffered that year was just horrible," Arlene said.

In 1991, when she was forty-four, she had neck surgery, which the neurosurgeon assured her would solve her problems. "After the operation, I didn't have the same kind of pain in my neck that I had had prior to the surgery, but I still had this widespread pain throughout the rest of my body, and I always felt like I had some form of the flu," Arlene said.

After her primary care doctor dismissed the ongoing symptoms as being emotionally based, Arlene went back to the neurosurgeon. This time he told her he thought she had fibromyalgia and he referred her to the rheumatologist—whom she has been with ever since.

"He has tried everything to help me," Arlene said. "He said one of the most difficult things to treat is fibromyalgia. You can look fine to the outside world, while you feel like you're one step away from keeling over."

Because Arlene lost feeling and dexterity in her hands, she no longer was able to work as a dental hygienist. When she applied for Social Security benefits, one of the government lawyers on her case told her, "Well, you're a woman; you're prone to these things." It took four years for her to get approved for disability benefits. When that finally happened, Arlene said, "I was very thankful for the help that I received."

After she stopped working, she became an active community volunteer in several programs, including tutoring disadvantaged children in reading. Over the years, she's learned to pace herself. To deal with the fatigue that is a common fibromyalgia symptom, she takes a short rest every afternoon. She tries to exercise five days a week and also meditates. But she admits that there are times when nothing works and "I'll put myself in a hot bath, and then I'll put myself in bed. And that's it. If that's what my body tells me I need, then that's what I do."

Because she also developed osteoarthritis and psoriatic arthritis, she's tried different medications, but she eventually decided that "the side effects were worse than the symptoms. . . . I try to stay away from medication."

Having other chronic conditions along with fibromyalgia is not uncommon, according to UCLA's Dr. Volkmann, who explained there are two types of fibromyalgia: primary and secondary. Primary means that a patient just has fibromyalgia, while secondary means she also has an autoimmune disorder.

"There may be two different things going on, even though they clinically appear the same. We think that when people have ongoing inflammation from an autoimmune disease for many years, they can eventually develop fibromyalgia," said Dr. Volkmann. "Every doctor is different in terms of how they treat it and how they view it. It's definitely still stigmatized."

The stress of not being believed, or of having symptoms dismissed or misdiagnosed, can make fibromyalgia and autoimmune symptoms worse. Dr. Bilstrom said that patients at Bingham Memorial's autoimmune center are encouraged to do relaxation techniques, such as meditation or yoga: "If you've been to fifteen doctors and everybody thinks you're a hypochondriac, or depressed, now you have these toxic emotions and toxic memories that are driving physical changes in the body. We have to disconnect those memories—because you're always going to remember this stuff—from causing adverse physical, biologic, and biochemical changes in the body."

In addition to relaxation techniques, Dr. Volkmann, a dance minor in college, stressed the importance of a regular exercise program. "Exercise is essential for managing fibromyalgia, as the symptoms can worsen the more sedentary a patient is. I typically recommend walking, water therapy and restorative or yin [gentle] yoga. All patients with autoimmune disease can benefit from physical activity," she said.

Autoimmune patients at Bingham Memorial meet with a social worker to see if they need help coping with the psychological aspects of their diseases. They also are connected with community groups that can offer support. "Patients may have so much pain, fatigue, and brain fog, they can hardly get the kids to school. Some people are barely hanging on," said Dr. Bilstrom.

Dr. Volkmann pointed out that sometimes even simple daily activities are challenging for patients dealing with pain and other debilitating symptoms. That is particularly true with chronic fatigue syndrome (CFS), another ailment that disproportionately affects women. Some 1 million Americans have the condition, for which there is no cure. Women are two to four times more likely than men to be afflicted.

The CDC estimates that only 20 percent of people with CFS are correctly diagnosed. The agency says a defining characteristic of the ailment is profound fatigue after physical or mental exertion that is not alleviated by rest or sleep.[18] Other common symptoms are trouble with concentration and memory. Sometimes, even activities like showering and getting dressed are challenging for patients.[19]

As with fibromyalgia, patients with CFS may be stigmatized for an ailment that cannot be identified with lab tests, explained Dr. Volkmann. A complication is that patients with CFS may be in agony but look fine to the outside world.

One of the most famous CFS patients is author Laura Hillenbrand, who has struggled with the ailment since 1987. She was a sophomore in college when she suddenly was blindsided by fever, dizziness, and nausea, which eventually forced her to leave school. As reported in a *New York Times* profile: "A string of doctors tried to convince her that the illness wasn't real—it was all in her imagination, they said, or maybe it was delayed puberty, or perhaps heartburn, or an eating disorder."[20]

Ms. Hillenbrand was mostly housebound for decades, struggling with terrible vertigo that made moving difficult. (Despite this, she wrote two best-selling and critically acclaimed books, *Seabiscuit* and *Unbroken*.) Ms. Hillenbrand expressed angst over what it was like to be so sick and to not be believed: "I was not taken seriously, and that was disastrous. If I'd gotten decent medical care to start out with—or at least emotional support, because I didn't get that either—could I have gotten better? Would I not be sick 27 years later?"[21]

In a 2016 interview with *Stanford Medicine*, Ms. Hillenbrand described CFS as a humiliating disease "because it isn't taken seriously. You are treated with terrible contempt, sometimes by your own family. . . . You start to feel like nothing because you're told that all the time."[22]

But this interview included the hopeful news that after decades of illness, Ms. Hillenbrand's health had improved somewhat. She had embarked on a new life in Oregon, even being able to take a cross-country road trip from Washington, DC, an experience she described as "wondrous. . . . I had been set free. I was not well. I *am* not well. I am always dealing with symptoms, but I was free enough to have that experience, to see America."[23]

Documentary filmmaker Jennifer Brea was diagnosed with chronic fatigue syndrome in 2012, after having her symptoms dismissed for more than a year. In 2017, when she was thirty-five, Ms. Brea turned her journey with the illness into the documentary *Unrest*. Thirty years after Hillenbrand struggled to get diagnosed, Ms. Brea went through much the same experience, illustrating how little had changed in attitudes. A *Wall Street Journal* article on the filmmaker recounted how doctors speculated that she was depressed, stressed out, or perhaps suffering from a vague psychological condition caused by some long-ago trauma. In the article Ms. Brea said that because women are more likely to be stricken with chronic fatigue syndrome, doctors are more apt to dismiss the condition or blame the patient.[24]

The sense of suffering forever is one of the hardest pills for women with chronic conditions to swallow (especially since there is no actual pill that can cure them). And they often feel that they are waging this battle on their own, without sympathy or support.

UCLA's Dr. Volkmann stressed that with chronic diseases, there's a deeply ingrained misunderstanding "that these diseases are all in the patient's head and that they can somehow fight their way through it on their own. In some cases, family members will blame the patient for being sick. They don't think anything is wrong with them. A lot of times these are relatively young women who otherwise look well. Looks can be very deceiving. I think the biggest misconception is that the patient is somehow fabricating their experience. These conditions have a major impact on their quality of life."

6

CRACKING THE CEILING

Neurosurgeon Dr. Frances Conley made headlines in 1991 when she resigned her professorship at Stanford University in protest over the appointment of an alleged sexual harasser as acting head of the neurosurgery department. (The doctor in question was accused of inappropriate behavior toward female doctors, nurses, and students.) In 1988 Dr. Conley had become the first woman in the United States to be a tenured full professor of neurosurgery at a medical school.[1] After she quit, the university press office put out a news release offering the medical school dean's opinion that Dr. Conley's decision to resign had nothing to do with "reported allegations of sexual harassment" on the part of its new neurosurgery chair, Dr. Gerald Silverberg, but instead was due to her disappointment over not being named chair herself.[2] In letters to newspapers, Dr. Conley described an oppressive environment in which Stanford medical school faculty included *Playboy* centerfolds in lectures and used sexist language. She said that women who protested these actions were labeled "too sensitive."[3]

A few weeks later Stanford University's president brought formal charges of professional misconduct and sexual harassment against another university doctor, a cardiologist who faced complaints from two female students.[4] (A historical side note: Former Yahoo! CEO Marissa Mayer decided when she was an eighteen-year-old Stanford University student to change her premed major because of these instances of sexual misconduct. As reported by the *San Francisco Chronicle*, Ms. Mayer told the 2017 annual Stanford Directors' College that the medical school scandals had a profound impact on her career path. She opted not to become a doctor but to instead study computer science, leading her on a path to Silicon Valley, where, ironically, sexual harassment abounds.)[5]

In response to the negative publicity after Dr. Conley's resignation, in 1992 Stanford formed a committee to investigate the harassment charges against Dr. Silverberg. After her allegations finally were taken seriously, Dr. Conley changed her mind about resigning and returned to Stanford. Less than a year later, the same dean who had expressed skepticism over Dr. Conley's allegations now declared that Dr. Silverberg had shown a troubling insensitivity to female staff members. Dr. Silverberg was removed as acting chair of the neurosurgery department, much to the consternation of some of his male colleagues.

In 1998 Dr. Conley created more waves for Stanford when she wrote about her years there in the male-dominated world of neurosurgery in her memoir, *Walking Out on the Boys*. This book and her speaking out against sexism are part of Dr. Conley's legacy. Equally important is the inspiration she provided to future female physicians. One of those doctors was neurosurgeon Dr. Linda Liau, who was in her early twenties when she entered Stanford's medical school. During her neurosurgery rotation, she met Dr. Conley, who at the time was conducting research on bacterial toxins as a way to treat brain tumors. "She served as a mentor as well as a role model. Having female role models in this field is very important, because if you don't see anybody else doing it, it's not quite as easy," said Dr. Liau, now an internationally renowned neurosurgeon and researcher and chair of the UCLA Department of Neurosurgery.

After being taught by Dr. Conley, Dr. Liau made up her mind to become a brain surgeon, even though female medical students then were advised that this specialty was too difficult a path for women. Dr. Liau learned at a young age not to shy away from challenges. Her parents, poor immigrants from Taiwan, stressed the importance of an education, and she excelled in academics. In third grade, she was pulled out of class one day and told that she had to take some tests. This went on for a week. She then was abruptly—and without any explanation—moved ahead two grades. (Later in life, she realized she had been given aptitude tests.) Dr. Liau was only sixteen when she graduated from high school, then headed to Brown University, where she double-majored in political science and biochemistry.

After graduating from Brown, she decided to attend medical school at a strong research university and set her sights on Stanford. But her parents could not afford the private school and told her she would have to pay for it herself. Trying to figure out a way to earn her tuition, she came up with the creative solution of getting her California real estate license. "I had turned eighteen, so I was old enough to get a license. I worked for Coldwell Banker that summer, and I was good at it," she recalled, smiling. "I sold two $500,000 houses at 3 percent commission and I was able to make my tuition for the first year."

After Stanford, Dr. Liau applied to the UCLA neurosurgery program. In the admissions interviews, she was asked if she planned to have children. "At the time I was twenty-three and not married and I wasn't thinking about children, and my answer was very honestly, 'No.' That was the right answer back then. If I didn't say that, I don't think I would have gotten into residency," Dr. Liau said, as we sat in her window-lined office above busy Westwood Boulevard on the UCLA campus. (It's safe to assume that male candidates were not queried about possible future offspring.)

At UCLA, Dr. Liau originally planned to focus on traumatic brain injury with two of the nation's leading experts, neurosurgeon Dr. Donald Becker and researcher Dr. David Hovda. But a tragedy in Dr. Liau's family changed the course of her career: Her mother was diagnosed with terminal breast cancer, which had metastasized throughout her body, including her brain. Years later, Dr. Liau's voice showed emotion as she talked about the impact of her mother's illness on her studies: "Even though they were able to control the cancer in other parts of body, they couldn't control the cancer going to the brain. That's when the topic of my research and my subspecialization in neurosurgery suddenly changed. . . . I really wanted to learn more about brain cancer and why cancers that go to the brain, either metastatic or primary cancers, are so difficult to treat. I needed to learn more about this so I could do research in this field and hopefully make an impact. What happened to my mom affected me so much. I went back to the lab and got my PhD in molecular neuroscience as it relates to cancer. During my residency, unfortunately, my mom passed away; I continued that particular topic of research."

Much of Dr. Liau's research has focused on immunotherapy as a weapon against brain cancer. One of the questions she has been trying to answer is why brain tumors frequently return even when surgeons successfully remove the original tumor: "The struggles that we have with treating the disease aren't necessarily how to get it out, but how to prevent it from coming back. I thought: Well, the best way to prevent things from happening is via your immune system. You prevent yourself from getting the flu because you go get a vaccine . . . so why can't you prevent brain cancer if you can vaccinate or mount an immune response against the cancer? That's been the gist of the biological/medical questions that I've been trying to answer for the past twenty-five years."

When Dr. Liau entered her neurosurgery residency at UCLA, she was the only woman in the program. "I'm actually only the second woman who's ever graduated in neurosurgery at UCLA. Even since then, we've only had one other. It's still a very male-dominated field." (In late 2017, when I met with Dr. Liau, there were three women residents and seventeen men in the neurosurgery program.)

When she was going through the program, Dr. Liau said she was referred to as "the little Oriental girl. . . . There was certainly much more of an explicit bias that this wasn't really what women should be doing. And even now there are implicit biases."

She met her husband, also a neurosurgeon, during the residency program. When she was thirty-one, they used the winter break to elope in Hawaii. After the honeymoon she began to feel ill, and at first she took it as a sign from the universe that maybe getting married was a mistake. Eventually, she realized that she was not receiving a cosmic message— she was pregnant. (Dr. Liau laughed when she told me this story, and I did, too—she clearly is brilliant, but just like so many of us did when we were young women, she misread the early signs of a first pregnancy.)

Dr. Liau went on to do something that none of her female mentors had been able to do—she became a mother to a son and then to a daughter. She said that the desire to have a family still can be a roadblock for women contemplating a career in neurosurgery because of the many years of education demanded by the specialty: "There is a hesitancy among some young women to go into a profession that really takes up so much of your time that it's very hard to have kids. That's certainly a consideration. . . . [I]t's a difficult decision to make."

She continued, "The women mentors that I had in neurosurgery, they never had children. Like Fran Conley, she never had kids. A lot of women neurosurgeons don't. There were women who went into the profession before me, but they had to choose."

In 2017 Dr. Liau was selected to lead UCLA's neurosurgery department, making her only the second of two female chairs of US university neurosurgery departments. (The first was Dr. Karin Muraszko at the University of Michigan in 2005.) And it's not just in neurosurgery that women have struggled to achieve leadership roles. Female physicians still have not been able to break through the glass ceiling in significant numbers to attain leadership positions in male-dominated specialties in academic medicine.[6]

In a paper on barriers women physicians face in academia, urologist Dr. Ashley C. Wietsma wrote that a key ingredient for success is having a mentor: "The presence of a mentor doubles a physician's chance of promotion. Without a significant amount of women in leadership positions, young female attendings, residents and medical students do not have role models to help guide their careers. This further perpetuates the problematic lack of females in academic leadership."[7]

The women physicians I spoke with all credited mentors with inspiring them, helping them to persevere, or just nudging them in the right direction. "The reason I enjoyed medical school so much related to the work I did, starting in my first year, with two female pediatricians in the division of pediatric endocrinology," said endocrinologist Dr. Connie Newman, adjunct professor, at NYU School of Medicine, part of NYU Langone Health and the 2017–2018 president of the American Medical Women's Association (AMWA). "I spent most of my extra time, when I was not in class, over the course of four years, going on rounds with them, attending a clinic, and doing research with their guidance. These were female role models."

Dr. Newman, who graduated from Weill Cornell Medical College in 1978, witnessed the ways in which female students were treated differently: "I read one of my friend's evaluations and it commented not as much on her performance but on the way she dressed."

Dr. Newman said she became active in AMWA so that she could mentor other women. She added that when she began her medical career, "you could start an academic career, but it was hard to get promoted higher than your entry position. I would have thought that this would be much better now. But research shows that it isn't. Women are now half of medical school students, but in academia very few of them reach the top."

She experienced this firsthand when she was an assistant professor on the tenure track. After spending eight years doing numerous studies and publishing important papers on mammary gland growth and development, she approached a senior faculty member: "I told him that I wanted to go up for a promotion, to become an associate professor with tenure. He was quite frankly shocked. He said, 'Why do you need to be promoted? You're married, your husband makes a lot of money.' I had to convince him. I basically pointed to the research that we did together. . . . He finally agreed that he would support me. If he hadn't, there was no way that I would have been promoted."

Dr. Martha Gulati, chief of cardiology at the University of Arizona College of Medicine–Phoenix, said there were male doctors who supported her and encouraged her to "dream of bigger things. . . . On my journey, there weren't many female role models for me when I was a cardiology fellow. But there were some excellent and outstanding male role models who never treated me differently because I was a woman."

Her most significant mentor was the late Dr. Morton Arnsdorf, a prominent cardiologist who was killed by a drunk driver in 2010. "He had such a profound influence on me. He was a great man and really ahead of his time, because he always tried to get women on the faculty," said Dr. Gulati, who nominated Dr. Arnsdorf for the American Heart Association's 2006 Women in Cardiology Mentoring Award, which recognizes individuals who mentor female cardiologists.[8]

Sometimes the inspiration to become a physician comes from unexpected sources. Internist Dr. Theresa Rohr-Kirchgraber, executive director of Indiana University's National Center of Excellence in Women's Health, was one of eight children; she got the idea to go into medicine while watching football with her father. "He was very into Notre Dame football, and the halftime show showed a baton twirler. I twirled baton for years and it was the desire to twirl in college and be on TV that encouraged me to go to college. Not the typical doctor story, but at least it got me thinking about college and education," she recalled.

It turned out that when she got to college, there was no time to twirl batons, because she had to work while in school. She had planned on becoming a nurse. With that in mind, and to earn money to pay for her education, she got a part-time job in an emergency room in Long Beach, California. There, a trauma nurse named Steven Wasserman urged her to rethink her career goals: "The summer before I was to start the nursing program, I was working in that hospital, Steven kept badgering me about why didn't I think about medical school. . . . I didn't know anybody who was a doctor, except for my own pediatrician. My parents had never gone to college; it just didn't seem like it was a possibility. That whole summer, Steven Wasserman—he was a pain—he would yell at me every time we worked together. He would point out a doctor and say, 'Look at that guy. You're smarter than he is.' He really gave me grief, but he also gave me a lot of confidence. I knew that if I switched and went premed, I would have three more years of undergrad, and I'd already put in three years. Or I could do one more year and be done. But he kept on my case and said, 'If you don't do this, you're going to regret it.' I ended up switching from nursing to chemistry premed."

I asked Dr. Rohr-Kirchgraber if she thought she would have become a doctor without Steven's encouragement. "I don't think that I would have," she said, "because I didn't have the confidence; I didn't know anybody who had done it."

Dr. Steven B. Wasserman, now a chiropractor in Los Alamitos, California, was touched and thrilled to hear that he had played a role in Dr. Rohr-Kirchgraber's decision to apply to medical school. "I just saw something in her," he said. "There's absolutely nothing wrong with the nursing profession; I think it's wonderful for the right person. But I thought she would make a great doctor. I saw leadership skills in her; I saw intelligence in her; she was able to take command. I saw so much potential."

Dr. Rohr-Kirchgraber ended up going to medical school at Cornell University, where she was inspired and mentored by Dr. Lila A. Wallis, a clinical professor of medicine who is considered a pioneering advocate for women's health as well as for female physicians.[9]

Born in 1921, Dr. Wallis became, in 1988, the only US physician to have board certifications in internal medicine, hematology, endocrinology, and metabolism. She is highly regarded as an authority on osteoporosis, estrogen replacement therapy, and menopause, and throughout her career she has fought for improvements in women's healthcare. She also promoted the idea that women should have a voice in their medical treatment.[10]

Among Dr. Wallis's many accomplishments was teaching doctors how to do painless breast and pelvic exams, something she learned from her own mentor, Dr. May Edward Chinn, who in 1926 became the first African American woman to graduate from the University and Bellevue Hospital Medical College in New York City (now NYC Health + Hospitals/Bellevue). Dr. Chinn also was the first Black woman to have an internship at Harlem Hospital. Dr. Chinn devoted fifty years to helping poor patients in Harlem, many of whom had advanced cancer that never had been treated. In the 1920s, Black physicians did not have admitting privileges at hospitals, so Dr. Chinn worked with other African American doctors in a private practice that served patients of color. As noted in an online biography: "Like all other black physicians in the New York area in the 1930s and 1940s, Dr. Chinn was barred from any association with the city's hospitals. She had tried to learn more about cancer after observing advanced terminal illness among her patients, but when she asked for research information about her patients from the city's hospital clinics, they refused. Chinn decided to accompany her patients to their clinic appointments, explaining that she was the patient's family physician. In so doing, she could learn more about biopsy technique while securing a firm diagnosis for her patients. Such resourcefulness typified Chinn's approach to the barriers she faced during her career."[11]

"IT ABSOLUTELY FILTERS DOWN TO PATIENT CARE"

I asked several prominent female doctors if they feel that the challenges facing women physicians in advancing in their careers ultimately affect patient care. "It absolutely filters down to patient care," said Dr. Rohr-Kirchgraber. "It's an unconscious bias. . . . You need some diversity at the highest levels, because that's what brings in different ideas; it brings in other ways of doing things. If everybody at the top all looks the same, that doesn't happen."

This is of particular concern for Black women, who may receive a double dose of prejudice—gender bias and racism—when they seek medical care. "With only 4 percent of all US physicians being African American and only 2 percent being African American women, it makes it a challenge, because you're not likely to be treated by somebody who looks like you or even understands what it means to be a black woman in this society," said Linda Goler Blount, president and CEO of the Black Women's Health Imperative.

Filmmaker Crystal R. Emery was so troubled by the lack of Black female physicians, she addressed the problem in her 2016 documentary, *Black Women in Medicine*.[12] In the film, she interviewed Dr. Jennifer

Ellis, then one of only six Black female cardiothoracic surgeons in the United States. As Ms. Emery wrote in a *Time* magazine essay, Dr. Ellis told her that "the further away your appearance is from TV's Marcus Welby, the harder it is for people to believe you're a doctor."[13]

Ms. Emery wrote that while making the documentary she learned that "minority doctors are more likely to provide care to minority, underserved, and disadvantaged communities, meaning their under-representation is of utmost concern. We all must challenge the status quo by replacing the false and debasing historical narrative regarding race, ethnicity and gender with positive, empowering images."[14]

Identical twins Dr. Brandi Jackson and Dr. Brittani Jackson launched a website in 2018, MedLikeMe.com, to help minority students pursue careers in medicine. Growing up, the girls often were the only African American students in their honors classes. Despite their academic success, they doubted themselves and had imposter syndrome, which they believe is common among women and minorities. Both attended Cornell University, where the thought of becoming doctors took hold after Brittani met a Black female physician for the first time. After attending medical school (Brittani went to the University of Michigan Medical School and Brandi attended Northwestern University Feinberg School of Medicine), the young doctors' goal was to work in an underserved community. Today, Dr. Brandi Jackson is the chief resident of psychiatry and Dr. Brittani Jackson is the chief resident of family medicine at the University of Illinois at Chicago.[15]

HARASSMENT AND OTHER BARRIERS

With the #MeToo movement revealing sexual harassment in nearly every industry, it was only a matter of time before medicine had its day of reckoning. A 1995 survey found that 52 percent of academic medical faculty women reported experiencing harassment.[16] In the decades since, the problem has not gone away. A 2018 months-long investigation by NBC News illustrated how harassment persists in medical settings. For example, surgeon Dr. Christina Jenkins experienced lewd comments from a male attending physician while she was in the middle of a complicated surgical procedure. She also was told by a male resident that he could make life easier for her if she had sex with him. Dr. Jenkins was one of a

dozen women who told the network about widespread inappropriate behavior in hospitals. [17]

The National Academies of Sciences, Engineering, and Medicine released a report in 2018 documenting how prevalent sexual harassment is
in academic life. Observed the advocacy group 500 Women Scientists:
"The authors of the report show how and why sexual harassment—and
the ignorance and disregard of it—is tightly woven into the fabric of
academia. This is not surprising to many of us who have experienced
harassment, but the sheer magnitude and universality of women's experiences is still astounding." [18]

Critical care physician Dr. Rana Awdish, director of the Pulmonary
Hypertension Program at Henry Ford Hospital in Detroit, said that when
she entered medical school in 1998, women were still in the minority and
sexual harassment was an ongoing issue. When I asked her if she had
encountered sexual harassment during her training, she responded emphatically: "Oh, absolutely! I literally don't know a single woman who
has not."

Dr. Awdish continued, "In many ways the #MeToo movement has
begun to reach medicine. Behavior that was tolerated, and almost
endorsed, is no longer. That bullying, the sexual harassment, the discrimination that every woman has faced in academic medicine, people are
being held to task for it now in a way that is allowing women to say, 'I
don't have to put up with this to have this job.'"

Cardiologist Dr. Alexandra Lucas wrote in an editorial that there is an
"illness" in the field of cardiology causing female physicians to be regarded as second-class citizens, which ultimately causes harm both to the
profession and to patients. [19] A survey examining quality-of-life issues
among cardiologists found that some 65 percent of women cardiologists
have experienced professional bias, including sexual discrimination or
harassment. [20] One of the cardiologists who worked on the survey, Dr.
Gulati, remembered when she was in medical school and was asked out
by a senior resident: "I didn't think that was a good idea, nor was I
interested. I said no very nicely. I wasn't rude; I just said, 'I'm busy as a
medical student; I don't have time.' I kind of made it all about work. And
he ultimately filled out my evaluation, and—surprise, surprise—I didn't
do so well."

More recently, she struggled with how to manage a colleague who has
a reputation as a harasser. "I haven't had any personal encounters with

him, but the point is I never allow myself to be in a room alone with him, or I make sure the door is open. Everyone warned me about him. You have these awkward situations. You might be a smaller person and you can't necessarily fight somebody off. . . . I do think it happens at lots of levels of medicine," said Dr. Gulati.

Clinical neuropsychologist Jill Brooks experienced sexual harassment when she was on the neurology and neurosurgery faculties at a New Jersey medical school. She and three other women—a neurologist, a nurse, and a ward clerk—who also were harassed by the same doctor filed complaints together. Initially they were discouraged from reporting the abuse and were told that the doctor could sue them for defamation of character. Nevertheless, the group persisted. In the end, the accused doctor was allowed to keep his position as chairman of the department and was required only to attend anger management classes.

In this kind of environment, where sexual harassment is either condoned or ignored, it's not surprising that some patients of university doctors suffer abuse. Perhaps the most infamous example of an abusive university doctor was that of Lawrence G. Nassar, who was found guilty in 2018 of molesting members of USA Gymnastics and lost his medical license. In addition to serving as the national team doctor, Nassar was a professor in the College of Osteopathic Medicine at Michigan State University. In both roles, he committed crimes against women for more than twenty years.[21] In addition to Olympic athletes, some of his victims were students and other girls and young women who were his patients at a university clinic. Not a gynecologist, Nassar employed supposed gynecologic "treatments" for sports-related injuries. He wrote a letter claiming that his touching of patients was appropriate medical care and that some victims' accounts were "fabricated. . . . The media convinced them that everything I did was wrong and bad. . . . Hell hath no fury like a woman scorned."[22]

One of Nassar's victims, Kentucky lawyer Rachael Denhollander, was fifteen years old when she was sexually abused by him. In 2016 she filed the first police complaint against him. She wrote that "the effort it took to move this case forward—especially as some called me an 'ambulance chaser' just 'looking for a payday'—often felt crushing. Yet all of it served as a reminder: These were the very cultural dynamics that had allowed Larry Nassar to remain in power."[23]

Another shocking example of abuse by a university physician took place at the University of Southern California, which was roiled by allegations in 2018 about longtime campus gynecologist George Tyndall. Nurses in the exam room said that Tyndall's comments to patients—and how he touched women—were inappropriate.[24] Many of his young patients had never been to a gynecologist before college; Tyndall (who lost his medical license in 2018) took advantage of their lack of knowledge about what constituted a normal gynecological exam. He used his position of power to humiliate, physically harm, sexually abuse, and photograph patients who trusted him. The nurses who worked with Tyndall reported him on numerous occasions to administrators, who did not take action until one fed-up nurse took her concerns to the campus rape crisis center. The *Los Angeles Times* won the 2019 Pulitzer Prize in Investigative Reporting for its groundbreaking reporting on Tyndall.

This was not the first physician scandal to rock USC. In 2017 a *Los Angeles Times* investigation revealed that medical school dean Carmen Puliafito, an ophthalmologist and prolific fundraiser for the school, had been leading a double life, including using illegal drugs with addicts and dealers, sometimes even on the same days that he saw patients.[25] Puliafito (who lost his medical license in 2018) was replaced as dean by Dr. Rohit Varma, who then was forced out when the *Los Angeles Times* prepared to report that he had sexually harassed a female fellow he supervised and had retaliated against her for refusing his advances.[26]

A CULTURE OF QUIET

When it comes to sexual harassment and assault, in the past there seemed to be a culture of quiet in the medical community, where doctors—especially those who generated significant income for their institutions—were protected, while female accusers either were not believed or were thrown under the bias bus. As reported in an extensive investigation by the *Atlanta Journal and Constitution*, numerous doctors accused of inappropriate behavior still kept their jobs. The series documented horrific cases of girls and women of all ages being assaulted by doctors from every specialty. The paper's investigation determined that when a physician is accused of sexual misconduct, hospitals or medical schools often look the other way or medical boards give offenders second chances.[27] A 2018 paper published by the Association of American Medical Colleges noted that while more women now achieve leadership roles in academic medicine, they still face sexual harassment and avoid reporting incidents because of a fear of retaliation.[28]

"I know it happens," said NYU's Dr. Newman, who started a closed Facebook group of more than one thousand medical students and doctors who attend or graduated from Wellesley College, her undergraduate alma mater. "People have written in about sexual harassment. It still occurs. It certainly occurred when I was in medical school. Not as blatantly as Harvey Weinstein, but there was some behavior that was just not appropriate. If someone is teaching you, they should not be propositioning you. Sometimes that did occur, but in my day, in the 1970s or 1980s, we didn't talk about it and we didn't go to the dean." Dr. Newman said that women still are afraid to report incidents of harassment "because they think that it might be held against them. There are fears of retaliation, which still exist."

Dr. Kimberly Templeton, a professor of orthopedic surgery at the University of Kansas Medical Center and past president (2016–2017) of AMWA, told me that some female medical students and doctors are worried that if they report inappropriate behavior, it may result in damaging repercussions both personally and professionally, especially if it is revealed that they filed the complaint. Women are not always convinced that reports will remain confidential. "The other concern is that they'll report it and nothing will be done," she said. "They think, *Why put yourself on the line if you think nothing is going to happen?* Abusers are typically serial abusers—they have engaged in this behavior for years and have gotten away with it. So if women see someone who demonstrates this sort of inappropriate behavior, and then hear the stories from women who have experienced similar harassing behavior in the past, often they assume that nothing will ever be done, either in terms of a specific offender or the culture of a system in general."

Dr. Templeton continued, "The idea that I try to emphasize to people is that sexual harassment has nothing to do with sex or sexual attraction—it is about maintaining the power differential. If you're in a field that is or has historically been primarily male and is run by men, and a man sees a woman starting to come up through the ranks in that field, he may feel threatened. Sexual harassment, in the broad expanse of how that is demonstrated, is his way of trying to reset the power structure as he thinks that it should be and to maintain the status quo."

"THIS IS WHAT A SURGEON LOOKS LIKE"

On April 3, 2017, the *New Yorker* featured a cover that caught the attention of female surgeons everywhere. The illustration, by artist Malika Favre, shows four female physicians in surgical gear standing under a bright operating room light, peering down at an unseen patient. As reported by *HuffPost*, the cover inspired female surgeons around the world to re-create the cover in photographs and to tweet out: #ILookLikeASurgeon. The *HuffPost* piece pointed out that female doctors in scrubs in a hospital typically are mistaken for nurses, while male medical students in scrubs are automatically assumed to be physicians.[29]

When 125 female surgeons convened in Ann Arbor, Michigan, in November 2017, the goal was to talk about how to overcome hurdles that prevent women from succeeding as surgeons. As reported in *General Surgery News*: "Many speakers spoke of the need for intentional efforts in recruitment, retention, compensation, negotiations and mentorship to raise the position of women in surgery, as well as that of surgeons from ethnic minorities or who are LGBTQ."[30]

When she decided to apply to orthopedic surgery residency, Dr. Templeton described herself as naive about the possible hurdles of gender bias: "I never considered that some fields could be almost exclusively male. I didn't have a mentor during medical school and attempted to guide my career on my own. Knowing what I was getting into, as well as having a mentor, would have helped significantly. I kept wondering, as I was going for my residency interviews, why there were so few women."

At one of her interviews, Dr. Templeton was told by a faculty member that they would not even consider admitting a woman because several years before, one of the female residents in another specialty had become pregnant during her training. When Dr. Templeton was accepted into an orthopedic residency in the late 1980s, she was the first and only woman in the program.

"I didn't really realize until I was accepted into a residency program that it was relatively tough for women to get into orthopedic surgery. It's a little easier now, but it's still very much a male-dominated field," Dr.

Templeton said. "I think there is still the myth that it requires a significant amount of strength to be able to do orthopedics. In fact, the most common thing that we do is talk with patients. And many of the procedures that we perform actually don't require a lot of strength but do require mental and physical stamina. There are some procedures that require strength, but those are the things that everyone, including men, may need assistance with, and you work together."

Only 13 percent of orthopedic surgeons are female, making it slightly better than neurosurgery, where 12 percent of all neurosurgery residents are female. A 2017 Harvard University paper found that gender bias decreases referrals to female surgeons, who are judged much more harshly than are male surgeons. The paper's author, Harvard researcher Heather Sarsons, noted that physicians increase referrals "more to a male surgeon than to a female surgeon after a good patient outcome but lower their referrals more to a female surgeon than a male surgeon after a bad outcome. Furthermore, a physician's experience with one female surgeon influences his or her referrals to other female surgeons in the same specialty. An experience with a male surgeon has no impact on a physician's behavior toward other male surgeons. These asymmetric responses imply that even if women are hired at the same rate as men, they receive fewer chances to show that they can be successful which could lead to lower promotion rates and wages."[31]

Despite a move by medical schools to increase the diversity of their students, women and minority physicians continue to be underrepresented in certain areas of medicine, especially surgical specialties. One study looking at whether gender bias discouraged women from pursuing surgery found that the majority of study participants reported experiencing gender-based discrimination during medical school, residency, and practice.[32]

Researchers found that women in academic surgery "receive less personal support and career advancement, as well as markedly lower salaries, despite practice settings, work hours and years of training. In fact, the percent of female leaders in academic surgery remains the lowest of all the academic medicine departments."[33]

A 2017 study by Doximity, an online social networking platform for US physicians, found there is a "stark" difference in how much women physicians earn compared with their male counterparts. The study reported that on average, women doctors earn 26.5 percent less than comparable male doctors and that there is no medical specialty in which women earn more than men. For example, female neurosurgeons typically earn $90,000 less, on average, per year.[34]

"In an hour I'm giving a lecture on gender and salary. It's still an issue, because women physicians get paid less than male physicians. Even though we've been told in the past, 'You don't really need to, because your husband is working or your husband's a doctor.' Well, you know what? Seventy-one percent of female physicians are the breadwinners in their families. We need to be making what we deserve and part of the discussion this afternoon is going to be about knowing what you're worth and asking for what you're worth," Dr. Rohr-Kirchgraber told me.

Sometimes it seems that female physicians take one step forward and two backward. For example, in gastroenterology, women have made significant progress in attaining fellowships and university positions. As reported by *Gastroenterology & Endoscopy News*, in 2017 the presidents of the four large national societies were women, yet female gastroenterologists still earn significantly less than male colleagues.[35] Medscape's 2017 survey of gastroenterologists' annual salaries reported that women earned an average of $308,000 while men earned $409,000, a difference of 28 percent.[36]

Cardiologist Dr. Gulati said that she left her prior university job after learning that her former male fellow, whom she mentored, was hired at her salary, despite the fact that she had twelve years' seniority: "When I called my boss out on it, he responded, 'Oh, we know what your husband earns; do you really need this to be about money?'" said Dr. Gulati. "I want to be paid what I'm worth. This has nothing to do with my husband; it has nothing to do with his income. It's about going to work every day and asking, 'Am I being rewarded for what I do?' It was insulting."

Even in the one area of medicine that is dominated by women— nursing—women still earn less than men. According to a 2015 study by the University of California, San Francisco, male registered nurses earn higher salaries than female nurses in equivalent jobs.[37]

The study noted that male registered nurses earn more than "female RNs across settings, specialties, and positions with no narrowing of the pay gap over time. . . . A salary gap by gender is especially important in nursing because this profession is the largest in health care and is predominantly female, affecting approximately 2.5 million women."[38]

Female nurses face other challenges as well. According to nurses.org, nurses face on-the-job sexual harassment, not only from some doctors but also from patients. An article by the investigative news organization Fair-Warning reported that despite forty-two states having penalties for assaulting nurses, hospitals typically don't report such violence.[39] The executive director of the Missouri Nurses Association said in a blog post that harassment—in the form of inappropriate jokes, comments, and touching—is common: "I suspect that if you ask nurses if they've been harassed by patients, a majority would say yes. Nearly every nurse will run into it at some time in their career."[40]

Nurses often do not get credit for the key role they play in patient care or in medical breakthroughs. A *New York Times* obituary for obstetrician Dr. William McBride reported that although he was credited with sounding the alarm about the sedative thalidomide and its link to devastating birth defects, it actually may have been nurse Pat Sparrow who initially alerted him to the drug's dangers.[41]

Based on their hands-on experiences and observations, nurses have devised inventions to improve conditions for patients and doctors, including a tube that allowed paralyzed veterans to feed themselves, different colored IV lines to reduce medical mistakes, and a garment designed to prevent surgeons from overheating in the operating room.[42]

Both female nurses and doctors feel they sometimes are not given the same level of respect as are men in medicine. It's not uncommon for female physicians to be called by their first names, or to be asked in meetings, "What do the girls think?" Dr. Gulati described this as demeaning: "We are not *girls*, we are women, we are physicians, we are your colleagues. . . . Not unlike many other professions, we're highly educated, we've worked hard to get where we are; some would argue we've had to work even harder than men to prove ourselves."

Female doctors have long bristled over being addressed by their first names at formal meetings, panel discussions, conferences, and grand rounds, while the male physicians are always called "Doctor." A group of Mayo Clinic doctors studied the issue and concluded that calling women by their first names instead of as "Doctor" has ramifications such as disrespect, marginalization, and discomfort.[43]

Internist Dr. Loren Rabinowitz wrote in the *New England Journal of Medicine* about an experience she had as the senior resident in an intensive care unit. The wife of a gravely ill patient called to speak with her husband's doctor—but she wasn't requesting Dr. Rabinowitz, who was in charge of the difficult case. Instead, the patient's spouse wanted to talk with a male intern who was the medical team's most junior doctor. Dr. Rabinowitz handed the phone to him, then was annoyed that he did not clarify that he was not, in fact, the doctor authorized to carry out the task the patient's family wanted. Dr. Rabinowitz also was annoyed at herself for not correcting the patient's misperception. But, as she pointed out "it seemed like the wrong time and place to advise an overwhelmed, soon-to-be-widow that she was engaging in sexism. On the other hand, acknowledging sexism's presence is necessary, even though doing so is nearly always uncomfortable. Broaching the topic is especially difficult in the emotionally fraught context of dealing with sick patients and their families. Next time, I hope I will find a way to be both kind and clear about my role in patient care."[44]

UCLA's Dr. Liau recounted that when she first started working as a resident, if she signed reports and recommendations including her first name, her notes often were ignored. When she switched to signing her directives "L. Liau," her recommendations were followed. She observed that for women just starting out, "in order to earn a certain level of respect and trust, it's almost like you have to pretend you're not a woman." Now that she is department chair, Dr. Liau always signs her full name.

But she still occasionally encounters implicit bias. She and a male colleague, an administrative officer, recently went to see a hospital CEO (whom they had previously not met) to discuss negotiations for emergency room coverage. When she and her colleague emerged from the elevator, the CEO rushed over and greeted the male administrator and shook his hand, without acknowledging Dr. Liau's presence or even making eye contact with her. "Then we walked into the board room and we went around and did our introductions. The CEO, realizing his error, was embarrassed. It was one of those automatic assumptions: If you're a small woman, you're not the department chair. If you're a big man, you are."

7

"THERE IS SOMEBODY SITTING HERE"

You might not expect a woman who had major surgeries for a serious heart condition and also for breast cancer—in the space of a year—to consider herself lucky. But Susan (not her real name) does indeed feel fortunate.

Her problems started while she was in her forties, when a gynecologist detected a heart murmur. Susan took that information to her internist, who monitored the murmur for several years and noticed over time that it gradually was getting worse. He then referred Susan to a cardiologist, where an echocardiogram revealed aortic valve stenosis, a narrowing of the valve in the large blood vessel that branches off the heart. This can reduce blood flow, forcing the heart to work harder and eventually leading to cardiac damage. In many cases, to avoid long-term heart problems, surgery is needed to repair or replace the valve.[1]

After her diagnosis, Susan's cardiologist told her that down the road she would require a valve replacement. The condition was monitored for five years, at which point the doctor said it was time to discuss scheduling surgery. The cardiologist explained the risks and benefits of different valve options, either a manufactured mechanical valve or one made from animal or human tissue. Ultimately, the decision was Susan's to make; she chose an artificial valve because these typically last longer. (Patients with this type of valve must take blood thinners for the rest of their lives to avoid blood clots.)

A year after Susan's successful heart surgery, she was diagnosed with breast cancer. Because she had a history of dense breast tissue and cysts, she had been seeing a specialist for ten years, getting regular MRIs and ultrasounds in addition to mammograms. "I knew that I had some problems. They were watching," said Susan. "They saw some calcification and they did a biopsy. That's when they saw there was invasive cancer."

Susan initially had a lumpectomy, with uncertain results. "They didn't get a clear margin on all the sides," she said, explaining that her doctors laid out possible remedies, including another lumpectomy, a mastectomy, radiation, and chemotherapy. Susan's cardiologist was brought into the discussion because some treatments could affect the new heart valve. "We went through all of the different options," she said. "I was part of the decision-making process."

Genetic testing revealed her cancer was a type that could spread faster than other forms of breast cancer.[2] Susan consulted with different specialists to determine the best course of therapy. Because abnormal cells were detected in both breasts, she decided to have a double mastectomy followed by reconstructive surgery. She chose not to have chemotherapy or radiation, instead having hormone therapy that would specifically target her cancer. Susan took these drugs for five years and is now cancer free.

Susan's case illustrates some aspects of the new thinking and progress that has been made in treating breast cancer. A groundbreaking trial, TAILORx, found that 70 percent of women with breast cancer can be treated with hormone therapy rather than chemotherapy, thereby avoiding often harsh side effects. (The study enrolled more than ten thousand women in the United States, Australia, Canada, Ireland, New Zealand, and Peru.)[3] One of the study's authors said the research findings upend the standard of care, meaning that thousands of women can avoid toxic treatment that would not help their prognosis.[4] Another study, published in 2018, found that women with advanced cases of aggressive "triple-negative" breast cancer—where patients typically have a poor survival rate—lived longer if they were given immunotherapy plus chemotherapy. Researchers hailed the study as a breakthrough treatment for this form of breast cancer.[5]

Looking back on her serious health challenges, Susan had nothing but praise for her medical teams. "I was lucky. I felt better having a good understanding of what was going on. That made me less nervous, and it made me feel more in control. I was able to talk to the doctors about all of the choices and decisions that had to be made. They listened to me," she said.

As Susan described the complicated conditions and treatments involved in her care, I was struck by how unusual her medical journey was, in that she was involved in every aspect of her treatment plans. Her questions were answered; her opinion mattered; her voice was heard. Susan's story also made me realize how important it is for patients to take an active role in their healthcare.

Making patients part of the decision-making process does not always happen, but it's essential, said Dr. Barbara Goff, director of the Division of Gynecologic Oncology at the University of Washington: "You need to provide the facts for patients. You are an adviser, but the patient's desires and own belief system need to be factored in. It's not a paternalistic decision."

In medical school, physicians traditionally have been taught to keep their own feelings in check and to interact with patients in a calm, dispassionate manner. The intent was to keep emotions from influencing a doctor's judgment. In a textbook this strategy might make sense, but in real-life medical settings, it sometimes results in patients thinking that physicians don't care about them.

Critical care physician Dr. Rana Awdish said that when she entered medical school in 1998 there was an ideal of clinical distance and reserve. To fit that profile, women students had to minimize their "attributes of empathy and nurturing, the things that are traditionally considered to be more female, because if we embodied them, then we didn't look like a doctor. To belong, we all adapted ourselves."

When she suffered her own catastrophic, nearly fatal health crisis, Dr. Awdish's vision of the doctor-patient relationship imploded. In her memoir *In Shock: My Journey from Death to Recovery and the Redemptive Power of Hope*, she observed that physicians "often enter the lives of patients on their absolute worst days. They meet without the benefit of social graces. Patients appear depersonalized in generic hospital uniforms. . . . [Patients] are doing their best to believe that they are worthy of the compassion and humility of a stranger. A humility that dictates that while we cannot possibly understand every patient's story perfectly, we can trust them to tell it, without imbuing it with our own biases. And when they tell their story, we can receive it, and bear witness to it. And in return for their willingness, however tenuous, to put their faith in us, we can do our best."[6]

At one point during her medical crisis, Dr. Awdish heard a physician yell, "She's trying to die on us." Dr. Awdish told me that moment jump-started a change in how she practiced medicine. While she understood that the emergency situation prompted the doctor's declaration, it nevertheless awakened her to the fact that medical practitioners sometimes see the patient-physician dynamic as adversarial, "that we feel we're in opposition, and how often as a doctor I had felt that but hadn't named it. . . . My training had biased me to believe that I was meant to act as the voice of medicine. What I realized from my illness is, that's not what our patients need. That wasn't what I needed from any of my physicians. What I needed was really somebody who was more willing to partner with me, and value their knowledge in equal proportion to how they valued my own knowledge of my body—not that medicine was the truth but that only really by combining both of our knowledge bases could we triangulate on the truth."

* * *

On more than one occasion, when something out-of-the-ordinary has taken place, I excitedly tell my husband about it, starting with, "You'll never guess what happened."

"What happened?" he wants to know.

I begin at the beginning: I left the house. I walked to the library. I bumped into Anne—it's been forever since I saw her. You won't believe what she said.

I can see my husband getting impatient—he wants me to cut to the chase. But, like many women, that's not how I tell a story. I take my time with the tale, with lots of important or amusing (in my mind, anyway) details, until finally I wend my way to the end.

In recounting a run-of-the-mill experience, there's nothing wrong with this approach (except for perhaps exasperating your partner). But in a medical setting, it's another story. Rather, it *should* be another kind of story. Better yet, it shouldn't be a story at all.

In my own medical crisis, had I done a poor job of telling my doctors about what was going on? The reality is, patients need to engage their doctors, hopefully inspiring them to think creatively about their condition. With that goal in mind, I now realize that the last thing you want to offer doctors is the kind of rambling account I tell my husband.

Instead, experts recommend coming to a medical appointment with an easy-to-digest executive summary of your problem. In a business setting, this kind of concise description is called an elevator speech—because it's supposed to be about as long as a typical elevator ride, a minute or less. In Hollywood, it's a log line, where you condense your pitch to a succinct synopsis that gives listeners the gist of the project while sparking their interest in you.

After that brief description of your problem, you should give very specific information of when and how symptoms occurred, and what you were doing when they happened. (Writing it out ahead of time on your phone or on index cards can help you from getting frazzled and forgetting key details.) Let's say you are seeking treatment for dizziness: When did the episode begin? Where were you? What were you doing? Did anything unusual happen? Okay, you got dizzy while you were getting dressed. Then you went downstairs. Did you have to hold on to the wall? Was the room spinning? All the specifics—the symptom details—are the things that matter and will help the doctor better evaluate your condition.

Experts also suggest trying to communicate health concerns without getting emotional. Obviously, dealing with an undiagnosed illness is upsetting—and it's maddening that physical symptoms in women often are brushed off as psychological—but it may help keep a doctor from jumping to that conclusion if you can remain matter-of-fact in relaying your medical information. If the doctor still seems dismissive, remember that you have the power to go elsewhere.

Dr. Marjorie Jenkins, an internist at Texas Tech University Health Sciences Center and the founding director and chief scientific officer for the Laura W. Bush Institute for Women's Health, said it's appropriate to consult with another doctor if you feel you aren't being listened to or heard: "If I took my car to the same mechanic five times and it still made the same noise every time, do you think I would go back to that mechanic? Women have to be healthcare consumers, meaning, if they don't get what they need in one practice, they need to go find a provider who will listen to their concerns and appreciate the fact that women know their bodies."

Dr. Jenkins added, "If a physician claims your physical symptoms of fatigue are due to depression and you know that's not the case, tell the doctor something along the lines of: 'I don't meet the criteria for depression. I'm not crying, I'm taking care of my family and I'm still doing everything I need to do. I don't believe that just because you haven't found an abnormality in the lab work, that means this is depression.'"

Once a doctor offers a diagnosis, patients should ask probing questions, such as: Is there anything else that this could this be? Are there other tests I should have? If the doctor refuses to engage in that conversation, again—find another doctor. If you are given a diagnosis and follow the prescribed plan but you fail to get better, don't assume it's the treatment that isn't working. It may be that the diagnosis simply was wrong.

Dr. Sami Saba, a neurologist at Lenox Hill Hospital in New York City, pointed out that a diagnosis—particularly one for vague symptoms with no clear abnormalities in testing—is an opinion. "That's all it is," said Dr. Saba. "If you get an opinion that you don't feel comfortable with, you can always seek another one. If you can get a personal recommendation for a doctor from family, friends, other physicians, that can be more helpful than just looking up somebody on the internet."

But even armed with a recommendation, Dr. Saba acknowledged that the process of finding a compatible doctor can be challenging for women: "How do they know which doctors are going to believe them, which doctors are going to put in the effort to figure out a complicated case? It's not easy."

A Harvard Health article offers tips on getting more out of a medical appointment, including sending your records to the doctor ahead of time and also bringing in the bottles of all the medications (both prescription and over-the-counter) you are taking, so there's no confusion about the strength and dose.[7] It's also a good idea to know what conditions grow on branches of your family tree, since many ailments have a genetic component.

When I interviewed her for a *Los Angeles Times* story on coping with a medical crisis, UCLA social worker Amy Madnick stressed the importance of having someone with you at appointments, especially after receiving a difficult diagnosis. "Don't try to do this alone," she advised, pointing out that when you are anxious, it's hard to assimilate new or overwhelming information. She suggested giving your support person a copy of the questions you want answered during the consult.[8]

If a doctor uses confusing medical jargon in discussing your case, you can be honest and say, "I don't understand." Ask the doctor if you can send follow-up questions via e-mail or if you can call. "I usually advise women to have a conversation with their physician and be inquisitive," said Dr. Alyson J. McGregor, director of the Division of Sex and Gender in Emergency Medicine at Brown University. "Ask whether the medication that they've been prescribed or whether the test that they're about to have is specific to discovering and treating these particular conditions in women. The doctor may not know that answer, but it will stimulate the doctor to think, *Oh, maybe I should look that up.* Physicians want to do well; if they are not aware of these differences, and it comes from the patient, they will embrace that understanding and new knowledge. So I always empower women to question their physicians and to have the dialogue."

It's also important for patients to be persistent. If you have multiple symptoms (as often happens with an autoimmune disease or other chronic conditions) consider consulting with different specialists who might offer a fresh perspective. If you need a referral, be up front with your primary care doctor, explaining that you'd like to get a second opinion and ask for a recommendation. A good doctor will not be offended or threatened by such a request. (But if your primary care doctor won't give you a referral, consider finding a new provider. You also can try going directly to your insurer to see if they can expedite an appointment with a specialist.)

Although consulting with "Dr. Google" sometimes is frowned upon, it can, in fact, be productive to conduct your own research on the internet before a medical appointment, sticking to respected sites such as the Mayo Clinic or the National Institutes of Health. There's nothing wrong with bringing your research results to your doctor, and saying, for example, "I'm concerned, because my symptoms sound like lupus."

If a particular symptom is worrying you, tell the doctor about it early in the appointment. Try to avoid a "doorknob" or "by the way" discussion—meaning, a problem you don't bring up until you are on your way out the door, either because it slipped your mind or because you were afraid to mention it. "By the way, I've been coughing for six weeks" is worth discussing up front, not as you're leaving the exam room.

In trying to get diagnosed, it's best not to underplay symptoms. Dr. McGregor urges women not to tell doctors, "'This is probably just nothing.' . . . I would like to remove that from the conversation." On that same theme, it's also important not to let our fears influence how we describe the symptoms. Nobody wants to face the prospect of a serious problem, but Dr. Awdish recommended being as honest as possible, allowing the "weight of the symptom to declare itself" without trying to make what is happening less or more than it is. Dr. Awdish pointed out that our feelings—whether anxiety or denial—can sway what happens in a doctor's office: "It's common to either worry that something represents the worst case, or you don't want it to be anything, so you minimize it. I don't think people realize how much physicians are really influenced by that editorializing. We want it to be nothing as much as you do. So if you say, 'Oh, yeah, this chest pain came on but I had had a big meal, it's kind of gone away,' that gives the doctor permission then to minimize it, too."

In my case, I now realize that I was too eager to accept two neurologists' responses when they assured me that nothing dire was going on. I didn't want to have a problem, so I was relieved to hear their nonchalant dismissal of my fears, which led to four years of being misdiagnosed. I like to think that going forward I would be much more assertive if faced with that situation and would demand to know: "What tests would you advise I have to rule out anything serious?"

Any woman facing surgery should ask additional questions, especially about the medical devices that may be used in the procedure. Amy Ziering, producer of the documentary *The Bleeding Edge*, an exposé about the medical device industry, recommends asking how other patients have fared with this device after two, three, or ten years. What is the device made of? Have these materials caused allergic or autoimmune reactions in patients? Has the device been tested on women? She also urges patients to inquire whether the surgeon receives payments from device companies. Ms. Ziering added: "The best protection patients have is to ask questions and do their own research. Know that your interests and those of the companies that stand to profit from your procedures are not wholly allied. So buyer beware."

These kinds of questions are not easy to ask. In addition, some women have the habit of putting themselves last and not wanting to bother people. In medicine, this can have disastrous consequences. "I didn't want to bother you, so I thought I'd wait it out" is something doctors hear, especially from older women. Women also may delay seeking medical help because they are busy taking care of other family members and figure their own health concerns can wait. And it's a sad reality that many people in this country cannot afford to seek medical care. Others avoid seeing doctors because of past negative experiences, adopting a philosophy of "what's the use?"

Based on her experience as a seriously ill patient, Dr. Awdish learned that not every doctor valued her voice, even when she was a colleague of the physicians treating her. She encourages women who feel dismissed to search until they find a physician who will listen. "There are people who will take symptoms seriously and dig until they find the cause. But it might not be the first person you encounter," said Dr. Awdish. "Don't be discouraged or think that somehow means there's nothing wrong or your symptoms are in your head."

Dr. Awdish pointed out that the insurance landscape and economic pressures have made it more challenging for physicians to interact with patients long enough to learn what is wrong. "So often, we don't have the amount of time we'd like to, to delve into things, which is why agenda setting is really important, to make the most of the encounter, and even to be willing to come back if not everything's been addressed," said Dr. Awdish.

She added that with all the technological advances there sometimes seems to be a disregard of the actual patient in favor of the virtual patient "who lives in the computer, who's a lot more manageable, who has all of their history and lab work and radiology there. I see it with young physicians who are getting the patient admission on the floor. They actually believe they know everything about the patient before they've ever met them, because they looked at everything in the computer. . . . And they have a plan of what they want to do, before they ever meet the patient. And that's terrifying."

Nurses often play a crucial role in making the medical team fully recognize what a patient is going through. Hospice nurse and author Theresa Brown wrote about how nurses can alert a medical team to subtle symptoms indicating that a patient is in danger: "Every nurse most likely knows the feeling. The patient's vital signs are just a little off. . . . But on paper she looks stable, so it's hard to get a doctor to listen, much less act." Ms. Brown wrote of the guilt she still carries with her over a patient who died years ago. As the on-duty nurse, Ms. Brown felt that the patient was having a sudden decline, but the rest of the medical team dismissed her concerns: "But I can promise myself that in the future, I will take any sense of urgency very seriously, document my concern and speak up. There's now solid evidence that when a nurse says she's got a bad feeling about a patient, the entire care team needs to listen."[9]

*　*　*　*　*　*

Dr. Awdish firmly believes that doctors cannot heal if they cannot empathize: "You can treat, but you can't heal. . . . Physicians are so attuned to
answer questions in a cognitive way, and they don't often realize that
questions are really a request for emotional connection."

Finding this kind of care can be challenging for patients who have
been mistreated and misunderstood. For example, it's only recently that
the medical profession has started to address the unique emotional and
physical challenges of patients who identify as gender diverse or transgender, who long have struggled to get appropriate medical care.[10] As
noted in a 2016 academic paper, "It has been well established by various
research projects that health disparities exist among the LGBTQIA+
community as a growing minority group. These biases are primarily
rooted in bias, stigma, discrimination and other social determinants of
health, rather than biological genetics or gender identity. The issues for
this population group exist not only within underrepresentation in clinical
trials, but also in day-to-day healthcare."[11]

In a moving essay, Dr. Laura Arrowsmith, who is transgender, wrote
of the time an emergency care physician refused to treat her for an infection related to her gender confirmation surgery: "Because so few physicians will treat this population, many transgender people have given up
trying to find medical care or are afraid to seek routine and emergency
care. . . . Unfortunately, information about the appropriate treatment for
transgender patients has not been taught in medical schools or postgradu-
ate programs until recently. . . . This has to change. No patient meeting a
physician for the first time should fear being denied care or given incorrect treatment. The expression on a caring professional's face should be
one of concern and interest, not a snarl of angry disgust."[12]

In some locales that situation has been improving as more specialized
healthcare centers open for gender-diverse patients, such as ones at
UCLA, Boston Medical Center, Johns Hopkins Hospital in Baltimore,
Mount Sinai Hospital in New York City, and Oregon Health & Science
University in Portland.[13] At the Vanderbilt University School of Medi-
cine in Nashville, students take specialized courses on LGBT healthcare.
The medical center has a unique program that offers transgender patients
a buddy to guide them through their care.[14] Still, many transgender pa-

tients fear or don't trust healthcare providers, finding the lack of empathy they often face throughout society is magnified in a medical setting.

At Stanford University, Dr. Donald A. Barr tries to instill in premed students the importance of empathy in all doctor-patient interactions: "When a person feels that their physician really understands them and values the perspective the patient brings to it, that leads to a greater sense of trust and satisfaction in the interaction with the physician."

It may also lead to a better health outcome. Dr. Barr said that when patients feel their doctor truly cares, they may be more apt to follow the medical directives, such as taking medication as prescribed and scheduling follow-up appointments. Dr. Barr encourages women to maintain and invest in a relationship with a primary care physician with whom they feel an empathetic connection, "following you as the whole person over the years, so you feel as though there is at least this one doctor who really understands you—even if you can't get the orthopedist to take your knee complaint seriously."

In his 2004 essay "A Time to Listen," Dr. Barr wrote about a life-changing experience he had with a new patient when he allowed her to talk to him for as long as she wanted, without interruption. The patient, a woman in her seventies, revealed that it was not her idea to see the doctor—she was only there because family and friends were worried about her cough. By the end of the day she had received a grave diagnosis of lung cancer. "This hasn't been a very good day for you, has it?" Dr. Barr gently asked her. To his surprise, the patient said that he shouldn't worry about her, because her life had been good. She patted Dr. Barr on the wrist and told him that this had been "the best doctor visit I've ever had. You're the only one who ever listened."[15]

I asked Dr. Barr how that experience changed the way he practiced medicine. He said that from then on, whenever he entered an exam room, he would remind himself to give patients plenty of time to talk about the problem that had brought them to him. "I would also do my best not to interrupt the patient's response until a 'reasonable' time had passed, and then only in a responsive context. . . . I emphasize this message to students when we are learning about the doctor-patient relationship."

Probably one of the greatest gifts a doctor can give a patient, in addition to carefully listening, is to be honest, even if the physician has no clue what might be wrong. Cardiac patient and advocate Starr Mirza, who suffered years of incorrect diagnoses as a child and teenager, observed:

"It is so much worse to make someone feel like they're crazy than to just say, 'Sorry, I don't know.' I've told doctors they need to learn how to say, 'I don't know.' Patients will respect you."

Best-selling author Laura Hillenbrand, who was misdiagnosed for years before learning she has chronic fatigue syndrome, recalled how she felt when a doctor honestly told her that he didn't know what was wrong with her, but that he believed she was very ill: "That took humility for him to say. I am so grateful for it. I walked out of there happy even though he said, 'I can't treat you. I don't know what to do for you.' But simply telling me, 'I respect you, and I have a limit to my understanding of disease,' was a beautiful thing."[16]

In our quest for better health, our most powerful weapon is the ability to ask questions, and to keep asking until we get answers that make sense. For those of us who grew up never grilling a doctor, advocating for ourselves can be challenging. But it's an essential skill that can be learned. Finding our voice in a medical setting is key to getting better care. Believing in ourselves and the truth of our symptoms—even if we are initially met with skepticism—may be the most important step we can take to fight for our own health. Finding doctors who value and trust our knowledge of our bodies, and who listen to us, is essential for healing.

Starr said she now doesn't hesitate to ask a doctor, "What can we both do to figure this out? What tests can I have? What can I do to make your job easier so you can diagnose me, so you can make me feel better? We're part of a team. You're treating a human being, not just a disease. I can honestly tell you that most of my doctors probably couldn't even tell you my hair color, because they never looked up from the chart. There is somebody sitting here."

AFTERWORD

This book originally was published just before the terms *COVID-19*, *surge*, and *quarantine* hijacked our daily vocabulary. As the tsunami of illness and death has swept across the globe, exhausted healthcare workers have been our heroes, putting their lives at risk to save the rest of us.

When I began writing this afterword, I hoped the pandemic might be in retreat. Unfortunately, that hasn't happened in most countries. With only a small percentage of the world population vaccinated against SARS-CoV-2, the virus that causes COVID-19, thousands of people continue to fall ill each day. While the disease may ebb and flow, many experts believe we will be dealing with it for a long time.[1]

The pandemic has magnified one of the fundamental points of the book: that disease affects men and women differently. An international study by Global Health 50/50, an organization working to advance gender equality in healthcare, found that differences "in women's and men's bodies due to their sex (biology) is playing a role in people's risk of illness and death due to COVID-19."[2]

The catastrophic health emergency has thrown light on systemic bias in medical care. As illustrated throughout the book, sick women long have struggled to be heard, believed, and treated. This pattern has persisted even during an international health crisis.

UCLA rheumatologist Dr. Elizabeth R. Volkmann, who discussed the challenges faced by women with autoimmune disease in chapter 5, has been disturbed by the experiences of some of her female patients with

COVID. Dr. Volkmann shared several alarming examples in which emergency room doctors dismissed women's life-threatening symptoms.

One of Dr. Volkmann's patients, who has rheumatoid arthritis and autoimmune lung disease, went to the ER when her COVID fever spiked. "The only care they provided was reassurance—even though she had been sick for fourteen days and was getting worse. They just sent her home without doing any imaging. A few days later she developed respiratory distress and was admitted to the ICU," said Dr. Volkmann. "A CT scan revealed that her lungs were full of inflammation. If they had done the scan when she was first sent to the ER, she would have been at a less severe stage of the disease. She fortunately survived, but it was a really scary time."

In contrast, after a male patient of Dr. Volkmann's became ill with COVID, he immediately was admitted to a hospital and then airlifted to a bigger medical facility. "I've had so many examples now of women being mistreated when I sent them to the ER. It's really troubling," said Dr. Volkmann.

Also disturbing is that COVID-19 has caused a new chronic illness, *long COVID*, which has afflicted four times as many females as males around the world. Some women (including younger ones with mild cases) have been left with lingering, debilitating illness.[3] In his book on the coronavirus, former White House senior adviser for COVID response Andy Slavitt tells the story of Thia, a documentary filmmaker in Northern California: "The aftermath of her bout with COVID-19 has been the most challenging time of her life. Today Thia suffers from extreme exhaustion, shortness of breath, ongoing heart palpitations, a painful rash that extends from her neck to her eyeballs, edema, life-threatening blood clots in her legs and both lungs, and numbness on one side of her body from a mild stroke."[4]

Most patients with long COVID are women between the ages of forty and sixty.[5] Common symptoms include headaches, shortness of breath, pain, nausea, fatigue, and cognitive issues. This pushes many women down the rabbit hole of multiple medical appointments and no answers.

NBC News reported on Ailsa Court of Oregon, who, four months after getting COVID-19, still experienced severe symptoms. One day the thirty-five-year-old felt so sick she feared a stroke. But an urgent care doctor rolled his eyes and brushed off her concerns. His reaction left Ailsa frustrated and angry: "I'm so ill and some people are telling me this is a figment of my imagination. It truly feels like a nightmare."[6]

"Nightmare" is a good way to describe what has happened to certain populations who have been hit particularly hard by the virus. Their well-being has been compromised because of societal issues—known as *social determinants of health*—including sexism, racism, violence, poverty, food instability, underlying medical conditions, and environmental factors. Mounting evidence reveals that communities of color have been shortchanged in testing and treatment. A 2020 analysis by the Brookings Institution found that in the United States, Black people died from CO-VID-19 at 3.6 times the rate of white people. For Latinos, it was 2.5 times the rate of whites.[7] A year later, the trend persisted: APM Research Lab reported that "Pacific Islander, Latino, Indigenous and Black Americans all have a COVID-19 death rate of *double* or more that of White and Asian Americans, who experience the lowest age-adjusted rates."[8]

US men have died at higher rates than have US women; however, death rates by gender fluctuate depending on the state, city, and neighborhood.[9] At the Harvard T.H. Chan School of Public Health, researchers and students in the GenderSci Lab have analyzed data from states' health departments. Tamara Rushovich, a PhD student in population health sciences, said that in some states "the mortality rate among men is almost double the rate among women. In other states, it's almost equal. That suggests there's probably other context—social factors, occupational exposures—that are influencing why the rates are varying between men and women, and that it's not only related to biological differences."[10]

There's no doubt that some tragic pandemic outcomes have been due to a fatal combination of sexism and racism. Horror stories of Black women with COVID being treated poorly are all too common. One haunting example is the tragedy that befell thirty-year-old Rana Zoe Mungin, a much-loved middle school teacher from Brooklyn. She was denied a COVID-19 test on two occasions, despite having a fever, cough, and asthma. As her condition worsened and an ambulance was called, an EMT speculated that Rana was having a panic attack and didn't want to transport her to an emergency room.[11] When she finally was admitted to a hospital, Rana was put on a ventilator for thirty days before being moved to a long-term care facility. She died on April 27, 2020.

Cardiologist Dr. Paula Johnson, president of Wellesley College (Rana's alma mater), called the disproportionate impact of COVID-19 on Black and Latino communities a "moral and systemic failure."[12]

The pandemic has taken a harsh toll on female healthcare workers, both physically and emotionally. During the first year of the virus, more than thirty-six hundred US medical workers died from COVID-19.[13] A study done eight months into the pandemic revealed that three-quarters of hospitalized US healthcare workers were women.[14] Many of those taken ill were nurses, who were exposed while delivering intense care and comfort to gravely ill patients—sometimes without adequate protective gear. By April 2021, a third of healthcare worker deaths were nurses, more than any other job group in medical settings.[15] (Nursing represents the biggest healthcare profession in the United States, with nearly 4 million registered nurses, triple the number of US physicians.[16] Approximately 90 percent of US nurses are female.) The professional association National Nurses United reported that the pandemic has had a "disproportionate impact on registered nurses of color."[17] A United Nations report noted that globally, women perform most support jobs in medical facilities, such as laundry and food service, making them more susceptible to COVID exposure.[18]

COVID-19 also has derailed the careers of some women in academic medical research, according to the National Academies of Sciences, Engineering, and Medicine. During the pandemic, many female scientists paused their work to focus on family issues, such as childcare and looking after elderly relatives.[19] This has hindered grants, studies, and clinical trials. Getting back on track is extremely difficult, said UCLA's Dr. Volkmann: "It's disproportionately affected women. When you have fewer women researchers, then you have fewer people caring about gender and sex issues. This could affect the future of medical research."

The erratic government response to the pandemic during the Trump administration jeopardized more than a million American women with the debilitating autoimmune disease lupus. This occurred after then-president Donald Trump (and Fox News) promoted the antimalaria drug hydroxychloroquine as a COVID-19 cure—despite experts saying there is no scientific evidence to support this claim.[20] Trump's bombast led to hoarding of the drug by healthy people, creating a shortage of the crucial lupus medication. (Ninety percent of lupus patients are women.)

After Trump hyped hydroxychloroquine, Maya Harris (younger sister of Biden administration vice president Kamala Harris) tweeted: "I have lupus. I haven't spoken publicly about it before now. But then coronavirus hit, killing black people at alarming rates & Trump unnecessarily put lupus patients—disproportionately black women—at higher risk."[21] (Lupus is two to three times more prevalent among women of color, who frequently experience life-threatening complications with the illness.)

Wendy Rodgers, a senior manager for community outreach with the Lupus Foundation of America, explained that hydroxychloroquine "helps to suppress the activity of the immune system, because with lupus our immune system is overactive. The majority of the medications we take are about quieting that down, to keep the disease from attacking our vital organs and causing damage and inflammation."

She said the misinformation about hydroxychloroquine created a scenario that was "devastating . . . some people couldn't access the medication at all. Others reduced their dosages or started taking it every other day. We really had to work overtime to advocate for the community. It was scary for many people."

Wendy shared her own courageous and harrowing journey with lupus in chapter 5. Her struggles to get an accurate diagnosis and effective treatment were worsened by encounters with sexism and racism. But Wendy persevered; after being on dialysis for nine years (lupus can damage the kidneys), she had a successful kidney transplant. During the pandemic, when her nephrologist told her she should get a COVID-19 vaccine, Wendy said she "celebrated. I was so happy to get vaccinated. I couldn't get there fast enough."

She is disappointed about ongoing efforts by the antivaccine community to dissuade people from getting inoculated: "That stems from fear and lack of knowledge about the benefits of a vaccine. Having lupus and having had a kidney transplant, I can't even tell you the number of vaccines I've been given, because my immune system is low. I've been able to live a positive and a healthy life because I've taken the precautions to protect myself. When people say they're not going to get vaccinated, it reminds me of somebody willing to play Russian roulette with their life."

Distrust of the vaccine is running high among women.[22] One contributing factor may be that they have been targeted by conspiracy proponents spreading the unproven theory that COVID vaccines cause infertility. This conjecture has gained international traction despite efforts by doctors to debunk the narrative.[23]

Concern over COVID-19 shots grew when thousands of women reported extreme postvaccination changes to their menstrual cycles, such as heavy bleeding that lasted for weeks. Many said their complaints were not taken seriously, nor were they warned about this possible side effect. In a call for studies on the issue, the National Institutes of Health observed that long-term consequences of the COVID vaccines on menstrual cycles "have not been investigated in a rigorous or systematic manner."[24] On August 30, 2021, NIH announced it was awarding one-year grants totaling $1.67 million to five institutions to research possible links between COVID vaccines and menstrual cycle changes.[25]

Endocrinologist Dr. Saralyn Mark,[26] lead COVID-19 physician for the American Medical Women's Association, explained that menstrual cycles can temporarily react to stress, infections, or vaccines, as do other vital signs in the body. She said there has been no reported evidence that any of the COVID-19 vaccines affect fertility.

"Everything we do in life is a risk-benefit analysis," said Dr. Mark. "When you look at the value of vaccines, at this point in time it is what we have to try to protect ourselves. With that said, it doesn't mean you negate side effects. You have to understand them and see what you can do to mitigate them."

About 80 percent of people who have reported side effects from the vaccines are female.[27] Dr. Mark, a former senior medical adviser to the US Department of Health and Human Services, NASA, and the White House, believes it is important to investigate whether women might do just as well with smaller doses of COVID vaccines, which potentially could decrease side effects while still offering effective protection. The CDC has been calling on scientists to analyze biological factors such as age, sex, and race when investigating vaccine responses.[28] However, as indicated in the book, getting researchers to follow such guidelines is a persistent problem. One paper noted that although "sex appears to be an important determinant of mortality risk and immunologic responses to COVID-19, currently registered clinical trials mostly omit sex as an explicit recruitment or analytical criterion."[29]

Initially, there was mixed messaging about COVID vaccines for pregnant women, but as of this writing, CDC and the American College of Obstetricians and Gynecologists are urging pregnant women to be vaccinated, noting that tens of thousands of expectant mothers already have safely been inoculated.[30] Evidence abounds that pregnant women who contract COVID-19 risk severe illness and death, as do their unborn babies.[31]

During 2020, the pandemic and the murder of George Floyd intersected and raised awareness of systemic bias on many fronts, including healthcare. On *PBS NewsHour*, journalist Yamiche Alcindor reported on discrimination faced by generations of Black women in their medical struggles. She told the disturbing story of Alie Streeter, who sought help for fainting episodes when she was in college. One doctor told the then twenty-two-year-old that she had tertiary syphilis, a disease that usually takes ten years to manifest symptoms. Alie explained to the physician that the diagnosis was not possible because "I wasn't having sex when I was twelve. She refused to believe me. She refused to believe that, at that point in my life, I'd only had one partner. And she just was adamant, would not look at any other options." Two years later, Alie was rushed to a hospital with frightening neurological symptoms and finally learned she has a complex type of migraine disease.[32]

There have been significant developments in other women's health issues, including menopause, long neglected in medical schools. Research published in *Neurology* in 2021 found a link between migraines and high blood pressure in postmenopausal women.[33] In another study, one of the few ever done to consider how menopause changes the brain, there was good news for women: Their brains can compensate for age-related declines. Lisa Mosconi, lead author of the study, told the *Wall Street Journal*, "Our study suggests that the brain has the ability to find a new normal after menopause in most women."[34]

In a *New York Times* essay, obstetrician and gynecologist Jen Gunter decried that menopause "has long been treated as a pre-death, a metamorphosis from a woman to a crone with her exit ticket already punched. . . . When women need help navigating their symptoms and the health implications of menopause, clear, non-sexist information and proven therapies should be available."[35]

There also was an important alert in breast cancer treatment, with the FDA issuing a safety advisory about robotically assisted mastectomy. The warning came after *Medscape Medical News* reported that clinical studies on the robotic devices lacked required FDA oversight. One safety concern was whether the robotic procedure leaves behind cancerous tissue.[36] Intuitive Surgical, which manufactures da Vinci robotic devices, is funding one of the suspect clinical trials. As noted in the introduction, one of this company's robotic surgery systems grievously harmed women during hysterectomies.[37]

On a different front, there has been growing recognition of the unique effects of traumatic brain injury in women. As pointed out in chapter 2, almost all concussion studies have focused on male athletes. But new research confirms that "female athletes are at significantly greater risk of a traumatic brain injury event than male athletes. They also fare worse after a concussion and take longer to recover. As researchers gather more data, the picture becomes steadily more alarming."[38] A 2021 study found that women are especially vulnerable to chronic post-concussion symptoms.[39]

It's encouraging that there is increasing acknowledgment of the harm caused by gender bias in women's healthcare. Dr. Janine Austin Clayton, director of the NIH Office of Research on Women's Health, offered this optimistic assessment: "Awareness of the problem is growing, as is an appreciation of the fact that women can have different diagnostic and treatment needs. I am hopeful that gender bias in health care will decrease over time."[40]

For now, many women in medical settings still struggle to be heard and believed. In her 2020 memoir, Sarah Ramey dubs one category of female patients as WOMI—women with a mysterious illness. Ramey has lived for years with severe illness that was dismissed by highly regarded doctors. She writes of sick women's "inability to find a physician to take their disease seriously . . . and the experience of hearing *But You Look Just Fine!* so often they could just cry."[41]

This scenario is very familiar to Wendy Rodgers: "With lupus, often you don't look sick. It's called the 'look good, feel bad' illness. It's also described as the 'cruel mystery' because typically it takes more than six years to be diagnosed. You have to do a lot of explaining and a lot of proving yourself, all while you're feeling bad. That's a big hurdle."

After so much overwhelming heartbreak and despair during these challenging times, I will end with a story that made me smile: In an Escondido, California, retirement community, breast cancer survivors have been using their stellar knitting expertise to help other women adjust to life after mastectomies. In 2018, when she was eighty-seven, textile designer Pat Anderson created Busters, breast-shaped bra inserts in all sizes knit from lightweight yarn and filled with removable microfiber pads. Two of Pat's friends, fellow knitters and breast cancer survivors, joined the project. The trio named themselves and their mission SBW: the Sisterhood of the Boobless Wonders. More than one thousand women have been given Busters, which have earned high praise for being much more comfortable than heavy, hot silicone prosthetics. Pat originally paid for the yarn and shipping costs herself, but then recipients surprised her by including generous checks with their thank-you notes.[42] When her inspiring story was featured on *PBS NewsHour* in 2021, Pat reflected on how grateful she and her friends were to be able to do this meaningful work: "The light, bright, cheerful colors help women remember that they are breast cancer survivors, not victims."[43]

Brava, ladies!

RESOURCES

SUPPORT AND ADVOCACY

American Autoimmune Related Diseases Association, www.aarda.org

American Cancer Society, www.cancer.org

American Heart Association's Go Red for Women (national movement to end heart disease and stroke in women), www.goredforwomen.org

American Myalgic Encephalomyelitis and Chronic Fatigue Syndrome Society, https://ammes.org

American Stroke Association, www.strokeassociation.org

Baby Quest Foundation (fertility treatment grants), https://babyquestfoundation.org

Black Women's Health Imperative, www.bwhi.org

Breast Cancer Prevention Partners, www.bcpp.org

Endometriosis Foundation of America, www.endofound.org

Fertility for Colored Girls, www.fertilityforcoloredgirls.org

GLAAD, Transgender Resources, www.glaad.org/transgender/resources

Golden Grain: Living a Fulfilled Life with Chronic Migraine, www.goldengraine.com

Hadassah, Coalition for Women's Health Equity, www.hadassah.org/advocate/coalition-for-womens-health.html

Heart Sisters: For Women Living with Heart Disease, https://myheartsisters.org

Jewish Free Loan Association, In Vitro Fertilization Loans, www.jfla. org/loan-programs/in-vitro-fertilization-loans

Lupus Foundation of America, www.lupus.org

Lymedisease.org, www.lymedisease.org

Med Like Me, info@medlikeme.com

National Brain Tumor Society, http://braintumor.org

National Breast Cancer Foundation, www.nationalbreastcancer.org

National Center for Transgender Equality, https://transequality.org

National CFIDS Foundation, www.ncf-net.org

National Fibromyalgia Association, www.fmaware.org

National Headache Foundation, www.headaches.org

National Heart, Lung, and Blood Institute, The Heart Truth, www. womenshealth.gov/heart-truth

National Multiple Sclerosis Society, www.nationalmssociety.org

National Ovarian Cancer Coalition, http://ovarian.org

PCOS Challenge: The National Polycystic Ovary Syndrome Association, www.pcoschallenge.org

Pink Concussions, www.pinkconcussions.com

Rheumatoid Arthritis Support Network, www.rheumatoidarthritis.org/ resources

Scleroderma Foundation, www.scleroderma.org

Society for Women's Health Research, https://swhr.org

Solve ME/CFS Initiative, https://solvecfs.org

Women against Alzheimer's, www.usagainstalzheimers.org/networks/ women

WomenHeart: The National Coalition for Women with Heart Disease, www.womenheart.org

NOTES

INTRODUCTION

1. "Sex Matters: Drugs Can Affect Sexes Differently," *60 Minutes*, February 9, 2014, www.cbsnews.com/news/sex-matters-drugs-can-affect-sexes-differently.

2. US General Accounting Office, "Drug Safety: Most Drugs Withdrawn in Recent Years Had Greater Health Risks for Women," January 19, 2001, www.gao.gov/products/GAO-01-286R.

3. Roni Caryn Rabin, "The Drug-Dose Gender Gap," *New York Times*, January 28, 2013, https://well.blogs.nytimes.com/2013/01/28/the-drug-dose-gender-gap.

4. Paula Johnson, MD, "When Does Medicine Leave Women Behind?" *TED Radio Hour*, February 10, 2017, www.npr.org/2017/02/10/514153036/when-does-medicine-leave-women-behind.

5. Roni Jacobson, "Psychotropic Drugs Affect Men and Women Differently," *Scientific American*, July 1, 2014, www.scientificamerican.com/article/psychotropic-drugs-affect-men-and-women-differently.

6. David M. Katz et al., "Preclinical Research in Rett Syndrome: Setting the Foundation for Translational Success," *Disease Models & Mechanisms* 5, no. 6 (November 2012), www.ncbi.nlm.nih.gov/pmc/articles/PMC3484856.

7. Rick Harrison, "A Drug for Women, Tested on Men," Women's Health Research at Yale, January 14, 2016, https://medicine.yale.edu/whr/news/article.aspx?id=11874.

8. US Food and Drug Administration, "100 Years of Protecting and Promoting Women's Health," www.fda.gov/forconsumers/byaudience/forwomen/ucm118458.htm.

9. Stacey Elin Rossi, *The Battle and Backlash Rage On: Why Feminism Cannot Be Obsolete* (Bloomington, IN: Xlibris, 2004), 240–41.

10. National Institute on Aging, National Institutes of Health, "BLSA History," www.nia.nih.gov/research/labs/blsa/history.

11. Steering Committee of the Physicians' Health Study Research Group, "Final Report on the Aspirin Component of the Ongoing Physicians' Health Study," *New England Journal of Medicine* 321 (July 20, 1989): 129–36, www.nejm.org/doi/full/10.1056/nejm198907203210301.

12. Fact Sheet, American Heart Association/American Stroke Association, "Cardiovascular Disease: Women's No. 1 Health Threat," https://www.heart.org/-/media/files/about-us/policy-research/fact-sheets/facts-cvd-womens-no-1-health threat.pdf.

13. National Institutes of Health, *NIH Guide for Grants and Contracts*, October 24, 1986, https://grants.nih.gov/grants/guide/historical/1986_10_24_Vol_15_No_22.pdf.

14. National Institutes of Health, "Bernadine Healy, M.D., Director, National Institutes of Health, April 9, 1991–June 30, 1993," *NIH Almanac*, March 3, 2017, www.nih.gov/about-nih/what-we-do/nih-almanac/bernadine-healy-md.

15. National Institutes of Health Revitalization Act of 1993, S.1, 103rd Congress (1993), www.congress.gov/bill/103rd-congress/senate-bill/1.

16. Janine Austin Clayton, "Applying the New SABV (Sex as a Biological Variable) Policy to Research and Clinical Care," *Physiology & Behavior* 187 (April 2018): 2–5, www.sciencedirect.com/science/article/pii/S0031938417302585.

17. Macaela MacKenzie, "Meet the Woman Helping to Fix the Gender Gap in Women's Health," *Forbes*, September 26, 2018, www.forbes.com/sites/macaelamackenzie/2018/09/26/meet-the-woman-helping-to-fix-the-gender-gap-in-womens-health/#1a010ee1dafc.

18. Erica L. Green, Katie Benner, and Robert Pear, "'Transgender' Could Be Defined out of Existence under Trump Administration," *New York Times*, October 21, 2018, www.nytimes.com/2018/10/21/us/politics/transgender-trump-administration-sex-definition.html.

19. "Sex and Gender: How Being Male or Female Can Affect Your Health," *NIH News in Health*, May 2016, https://newsinhealth.nih.gov/2016/05/sex-gender.

20. T. M. Wizeman and M. Pardue, ed., *Exploring the Biological Contributions to Human Health: Does Sex Matter?* (Washington, DC: National Academies Press, 2001), www.ncbi.nlm.nih.gov/books/NBK222294.

21. Ibid.

22. Johnson, "When Does Medicine Leave Women Behind?"

23. "Sex Matters: Drugs Can Affect Sexes Differently," *60 Minutes*.

24. "Women Remain Underrepresented in Medical Science, New Report Says," George Washington Public Health, March 3, 2014, https://publichealth. gwu.edu/content/women-remain-underrepresented-medical-science-new-report-says.

25. Janine A. Clayton and Francis S. Collins, "Policy: NIH to Balance Sex in Cell and Animal Studies," *Nature*, May 14, 2014, www.nature.com/news/policy-nih-to-balance-sex-in-cell-and-animal-studies-1.15195.

26. Charles Ornstein and Katie Thomas, "Top Cancer Researcher Fails to Disclose Corporate Financial Ties in Major Research Journals," ProPublica, September 8, 2018, www.propublica.org/article/doctor-jose-baselga-cancer-researcher-corporate-financial-ties.

27. Ken Jaworowski, "Review: In 'The Bleeding Edge,' Victims of Medical Devices," *New York Times*, July 26, 2018, www.nytimes.com/2018/07/26/movies/bleeding-edge-review-medical-devices.html.

28. Amy Martyn, "The Human Tragedy of Poorly Regulated Medical Devices Gets the Spotlight in a Netflix Film," ConsumerAffairs, July 27, 2018, www. consumeraffairs.com/news/the-human-tragedy-of-poorly-regulated-medical-devices-gets-the-spotlight-in-a-netflix-film-072718.html.

29. Ann M. Miller, PhD, "Gender Bias and the Ongoing Need to Acknowledge Women's Pain," *Practical Pain Management* 18, no. 5 (August 7, 2018), www.practicalpainmanagement.com/gender-bias-ongoing-need-acknowledge-women-pain.

30. Diane E. Hoffmann and Anita J. Tarzian, "The Girl Who Cried Pain: A Bias against Women in the Treatment of Pain." *Journal of Law, Medicine & Ethics* 29 (2001): 13–27, https://digitalcommons.law.umaryland.edu/cgi/viewcontent.cgi?article=1144&context=fac_pubs.

31. Alzheimer's Association, "Women and Alzheimer's Disease: A Global Epidemic," *National Women's Health Network Newsletter*, May/June 2015, www.nwhn.org/women-and-alzheimers-disease-a-global-epidemic.

32. Gayatri Devi, MD, *The Spectrum of Hope: An Optimistic and New Approach to Alzheimer's Disease and Other Dementias* (New York: Workman, 2017), 129–33.

33. Ibid.

34. Julia Reed, "The Gospel according to Oprah," *Wall Street Journal*, February 12, 2018, www.wsj.com/articles/the-gospel-according-to-oprah-1517918139.

35. Robert Pearl, MD, "How We Can Save 500,000 Lives in 2019 without Even Trying Hard," *Los Angeles Times*, December 27, 2018, www.latimes.com/opinion/op-ed/la-oe-pearl-optimism-health-20181227-story.html.

36. Vanessa McCains, "Johns Hopkins Study Suggests Medical Errors Are Third-Leading Cause of Death in U.S.," *Johns Hopkins Magazine*, May 3, 2016, https://hub.jhu.edu/2016/05/03/medical-errors-third-leading-cause-of-death.

37. Sami Saba, MD, "Dismissing Disease," letter to the editor, *New Yorker*, June 18, 2018, www.newyorker.com/magazine/2018/06/18/letters-from-the-june-18-2018-issue.

38. Maia Szalavitz, "Autism—It's Different in Girls," *Scientific American*, March 1, 2016, www.scientificamerican.com/article/autism-it-s-different-in-girls.

39. Alanna Weissman, "How Doctors Fail Women Who Don't Want Children," *New York Times*, November 30, 2017, www.nytimes.com/2017/11/30/sunday-review/women-sterilization-children-doctors.html.

40. Katherine Maher, "Wikipedia Mirrors the World's Gender Biases, It Doesn't Cause Them," *Los Angeles Times*, October 18, 2018, www.latimes.com/opinion/op-ed/la-oe-maher-wikipedia-gender-bias-20181018-story.html.

41. Hilde Hall, "My Pharmacist Humiliated Me When He Refused to Fill My Hormone Prescription," *Speak Freely* (blog), www.aclu.org/blog/lgbt-rights/transgender-rights/my-pharmacist-humiliated-me-when-he-refused-fill-my-hormone.

42. CBS News, "Arizona Pharmacist Refuses to Fill Woman's Prescription to End Pregnancy," June 25, 2018, www.cbsnews.com/news/arizona-pharmacist-refuses-to-fill-womans-prescription-to-end-pregnancy.

43. Oath of a Pharmacist, American Pharmacists Association, www.pharmacist.com/oath-pharmacist.

44. Chris Matthews, "Donald Trump Advocates Punishment for Abortion," *Hardball*, March 30, 2016, www.nbcnews.com/meet-the-press/video/trump-s-hazy-stance-on-abortion-punishment-655457859717.

45. Lynn M. Paltrow, "Life after Roe," *New York Times*, September 1, 2018, www.nytimes.com/2018/09/01/opinion/sunday/brett-kavanaugh-roe-abortion.html.

46. Kim Brooks, "America Is Blaming Pregnant Women for Their Own Deaths," *New York Times*, November 16, 2018, www.nytimes.com/2018/11/16/opinion/sunday/maternal-mortality-rates.html.

47. Nina Liss-Schultz, "The Woman Who Spent 3 Years in Prison for the Death of Her Fetus Just Got Out," *Mother Jones*, September 1, 2016, www.motherjones.com/politics/2016/09/woman-convicted-death-her-fetus-walks-free.

48. Katha Pollitt, "Mike Pence Might Be Even Worse for Women Than Donald Trump Is," *Nation*, July 21, 2016, www.thenation.com/article/trumps-vice-presidential-pick-might-be-even-worse-for-women-than-he-is.

49. Scott W. Stern, *The Trials of Nina McCall: Sex, Surveillance, and the Decades-Long Government Plan to Imprison "Promiscuous" Women* (Boston: Beacon Press, 2018), 5.

50. Jill Filipovic, "The All-Male Photo Op Isn't a Gaffe. It's a Strategy." *New York Times*, March 27, 2017, www.nytimes.com/2017/03/27/opinion/the-all-male-photo-op-isnt-a-gaffe-its-a-strategy.html.

51. "Women Are Watching," editorial, *New York Times*, September 28, 2018, www.nytimes.com/2018/09/28/opinion/brett-kavanaugh-jeff-flake-gop-women.html.

52. Sascha Cohen, "Breast Cancer Is Political. Tie That up in Your Pink Ribbon," *Los Angeles Times*, October 1, 2018, www.latimes.com/opinion/op-ed/la-oe-cohen-breast-cancer-is-political-20181001-story.html.

53. Gail Collins, "What It All Meant," *New York Times*, October 5, 2018, www.nytimes.com/2018/10/05/opinion/brett-kavanaugh-senate-susan-collins.html.

54. Kim Hutcherson, "CDC: Sex Assault Survivors Face Long-Term Affects." WILX 10, October 3, 2018, https://www.wilx.com/content/news/CDC-Sex-assault-survivors-face-long-term-affects-495116411.html.

55. Rebecca C. Thurston, PhD, et al., "Association of Sexual Harassment and Sexual Assault with Midlife Women's Mental and Physical Health," *JAMA Internal Medicine* 179, no. 1 (2019), https://jamanetwork.com/journals/jamainternalmedicine/fullarticle/2705688.

56. Nellie Bowles, "How to Fix Your Sad and Sluggish Sperm," *New York Times*, July 25, 2018, www.nytimes.com/2018/07/25/style/sperm-count.html.

57. CBS News, "Rebecca Traister on the Power of Women's (and Men's) Anger," September 30, 2018, www.cbsnews.com/news/rebecca-traister-on-the-power-of-womens-and-mens-anger.

58. Emily Dwass, "The 'It's All in Your Head' Diagnosis Is Still a Danger to Women's Health," *Los Angeles Times*, July 26, 2017, www.latimes.com/opinion/op-ed/la-oe-dwass-gender-bias-medicine-20170726-story.html.

59. Emily Dwass, "At Death's Door, Mercifully Blocked by an Ace E.R. Team," *New York Times*, September 26, 2006, www.nytimes.com/2006/09/26/health/at-deaths-door-mercifully-blocked-by-an-ace-er-team.html.

60. Johnson, "When Does Medicine Leave Women Behind?"

1. ALL IN MY HEAD

1. Emily Dwass, "A New Twist in Healthcare Billing: The 'Facility Fee,'" *Los Angeles Times*, December 21, 2009, http://articles.latimes.com/2009/dec/21/health/la-he-myturn21-2009dec21.

2. Emily Dwass, "In a Swoon," *Los Angeles Times*, March 5, 2007, http://articles.latimes.com/2007/mar/05/health/he-better5.

3. Medinsight Research Institute, "Study Raises Questions about the Safety of MRI Contrast Agent; Authors Call for FDA Action," EurekAlert! April 6, 2016, www.eurekalert.org/pub_releases/2016-04/mri-srq040616.php.

2. ALL IN HER HEAD

1. Steve Millburg, "Radiologist Wins Suit over Missed Aneurysm," *Highlights in Radiology*, February 2, 2011, www.radiologydaily.com/daily/diagnostic-imaging/radiologist-wins-suit-over-missed-aneurysm/.

2. Emily Dwass, "The Brain Tumor Is Benign, but Threats Remain," *New York Times*, April 27, 2015, https://well.blogs.nytimes.com/2015/04/27/the-brain-tumor-is-benign-but-threats-remain.

3. Ibid.

4. Rabbi Julian Sinclair, "Machatonim," *Jewish Chronicle*, March 6, 2009, www.thejc.com/judaism/jewish-words/machatonim-1.8109.

5. Gayatri Devi, MD, *The Spectrum of Hope: An Optimistic and New Approach to Alzheimer's Disease and Other Dementias* (New York: Workman, 2017), 135.

6. Mayo Clinic, "Stroke: Overview," www.mayoclinic.org/diseases-conditions/stroke/symptoms-causes/syc-20350113.

7. Alec Pawlukiewicz et al., "Posterior Circulation Strokes and Dizziness: Pearls and Pitfalls." *emDocs* (blog), March 15, 2017, www.emdocs.net/posterior-circulation-strokes-dizziness-pearls-pitfalls.

8. National Stroke Association, "Stroke Treatments," www.stroke.org/we-can-help/survivors/just-experienced-stroke/stroke-treatments.

9. National Institute of Neurological Disorders and Stroke rt-PA Study Group, "Tissue Plasminogen Activator for Acute Ischemic Stroke," *New England Journal of Medicine* 333 (1995): 1581–88, www.nejm.org/doi/full/10.1056/NEJM199512143332401?emp=marcomdel&.

10. Gina Kolata, "For Many Strokes, There's an Effective Treatment. Why Aren't Some Doctors Offering It?" *New York Times*, March 26, 2018, www.nytimes.com/2018/03/26/health/stroke-clot-buster.html.

11. American Heart Association, "Many Stroke Patients Do Not Receive Life-Saving Therapy," AHA/ASA Newsroom, February 23, 2017, https://newsroom.heart.org/news/many-stroke-patients-do-not-receive-life-saving-therapy.

12. Lokesh Bathala, "A Visit to the Stroke Belt of the United States," *Journal of Neurosciences in Rural Practice* 3, no. 3 (September–December 2012): 426–28, www.ncbi.nlm.nih.gov/pmc/articles/PMC3505364.

13. Jeffrey L. Saver, "Time Is Brain—Quantified." *Stroke* 37, no. 1 (January 2006): 263–66, www.ncbi.nlm.nih.gov/pubmed/16339467.

14. Centers for Disease Control and Prevention, "Stroke Facts," www.cdc.gov/stroke/facts.htm.

15. Centers for Disease Control and Prevention, "Leading Causes of Death (LCOD) by Race/Ethnicity, All Females—United States, 2014," www.cdc.gov/women/lcod/2014/race-ethnicity/index.htm.

16. Eliza C. Miller et al., "Infections and Risk of Peripartum Stroke during Delivery Admissions," *Stroke* 49 (2018), www.ahajournals.org/doi/10.1161/STROKEAHA.118.020628.

17. Kathy Webster, "Living Well with AFib," WomenHeart, August 27, 2018, https://www.womenheart.org/living-well-with-afib/.

18. Thomas M. Burton, "A Breakthrough Stroke Treatment Can Save Lives—If It's Available." *Wall Street Journal*, February 6, 2018, www.wsj.com/articles/a-treatment-is-revolutionizing-stroke-carebut-not-everyone-receives-it-1517933226.

19. Ibid.

20. Thomas M. Burton, "Hospitals Rush to Offer New Stroke Treatment," *Wall Street Journal*, December 26, 2018, www.wsj.com/articles/hospitals-rush-to-offer-new-stroke-treatment-11545836920.

21. David Newman-Toker et al., "Missed Diagnosis of Stroke in the Emergency Department: A Cross-sectional Analysis of a Large Population-Based Sample," *Diagnosis* 1, no. 2 (June 2014): 155–66, www.ncbi.nlm.nih.gov/pmc/articles/PMC5361750.

22. Dwass, "The Brain Tumor Is Benign, but Threats Remain."

23. Liz McNeil, "Cindy McCain's Secret Struggle with Migraines," *People*, September 2, 2009, http://people.com/celebrity/cindy-mccains-secret-struggle-with-migraines.

24. The Reliable Source, "Cindy McCain's Long Battle Inspires New Campaign," *Washington Post*, June 27, 2013, www.washingtonpost.com/news/reliable-source/wp/2013/06/27/cindy-mccain-launches-campaign-for-migraine-research.

25. "Migraine and Headache—Ask Dr. Ailani," MedStar Georgetown University Hospital, August 22, 2017, www.youtube.com/watch?v=a44I8pPSLeE.

26. RC Burch et al., "The Prevalence and Burden of Migraine and Severe Headache in the United States: Updated Statistics from Government Health Surveillance Studies," *Headache* 55, no. 1 (January 2015): 21–34, www.ncbi.nlm.nih.gov/pubmed/25600719.

27. Society for Women's Health Research, "Speeding Progress in Migraine Requires Unraveling Sex Differences," August 28, 2018, https://swhr.org/speeding-progress-in-migraine-requires-unraveling-sex-differences.

28. Rachel A. Schroeder et al., "Sex and Gender Differences in Migraine—Evaluating Knowledge Gaps," *Journal of Women's Health* 27, no. 8 (2018), www.liebertpub.com/doi/full/10.1089/jwh.2018.7274.

29. Jane E. Brody, "Giving Migraine Treatments the Best Chance," *New York Times*, September 18, 2017, www.nytimes.com/2017/09/18/well/giving-migraine-treatments-the-best-chance.html.

30. William B. Young, MD, FAHS, FAAN, "The Stigma of Migraine," *Practical Neurology*, February 2018, http://practicalneurology.com/2018/02/the-stigma-of-migraine.

31. American Society of Anesthesiologists, "Ketamine May Help Treat Migraine Pain Unresponsive to Other Therapies," *ScienceDaily*, October 21, 2017, www.sciencedaily.com/releases/2017/10/171021143928.htm.

32. Jaime Rosenberg, "American Headache Society Includes CGRP Inhibitors in Updated Consensus Statement," AJMC Newsroom, January 14, 2019, https://www.ajmc.com/newsroom/american-headache-society-includes-cgrp-inhibitors-in-updated-consensus-statement.

33. National Institute of Neurological Disorders and Stroke, National Institutes of Health, "Hemicrania Continua Information Page," www.ninds.nih.gov/Disorders/All-Disorders/Hemicrania-Continua-Information-Page.

34. Young, "The Stigma of Migraine."

35. Pooja Puvvadi et al., "Diagnostic Delay of Chronic Migraine and Medication-Overuse Headache in University-Based Headache Clinic (P3.135)," *Neurology* 90, no 15 supp. (April 9, 2018), http://n.neurology.org/content/90/15_Supplement/P3.135.

36. Gloria A. Bachmann, MD, et al., "Concussion in Women: Short- and Long-Term Health Implications," *Obstetrics & Gynecology*, May 2015, https://journals.lww.com/greenjournal/Abstract/2015/05001/Concussion_in_Women_Short_and_Long_Term_Health.87.aspx.

37. University of California, San Francisco, "New MRI Method Aids Long-term Concussion Prognosis," *ScienceDaily*, January 24, 2017, www.sciencedaily.com/releases/2017/01/170124140743.htm.

38. Susan Pinker, "The Perilous Aftermath of a Simple Concussion," *Wall Street Journal*, April 6, 2016, www.wsj.com/articles/the-perilous-aftermath-of-a-simple-concussion-1459963724.

3. VOICES NOT HEARD

1. Central Park Conservancy, Official Caretakers of Central Park, www. centralparknyc.org/things-to-see-and-do/attractions/dr-j-marion-sims.html.

2. Kate Grant, "Why Do a Million Women Still Suffer the Treatable Condition of Fistula?" *Guardian* (UK), May 23, 2016, www.theguardian.com/global-development-professionals-network/2016/may/23/why-do-a-million-women-still-suffer-the-treatable-condition-of-fistula.

3. DeNeen L. Brown, "A Surgeon Experimented on Slave Women without Anesthesia. Now His Statues Are under Attack," *Washington Post*, August 29, 2017, www.washingtonpost.com/news/retropolis/wp/2017/08/29/a-surgeon-experimented-on-slave-women-without-anesthesia-now-his-statues-are-under-attack.

4. Sarah Zhang, "The Surgeon Who Experimented on Slaves," *Atlantic*, April 18, 2018, www.theatlantic.com/health/archive/2018/04/j-marion-sims/558248.

5. Jennifer Gerson Uffalussy, "The Cost of IVF: 4 Things I Learned While Battling Infertility." *Forbes*, February 6, 2014, www.forbes.com/sites/learnvest/2014/02/06/the-cost-of-ivf-4-things-i-learned-while-battling-infertility.

6. Fertility Within Reach, "Grant & Discount Programs," www. fertilitywithinreach.org/financial-assitance/grant-assitance.

7. Shelley Skuster, "The Truth about Getting Pregnant after Adoption," Adoption.com, October 6, 2015, https://adoption.com/truth-about-getting-pregnant-after-adoption.

8. "The psychological impact of infertility and its treatment," *Harvard Mental Health Letter*, May 2009, www.health.harvard.edu/newsletter_article/The-psychological-impact-of-infertility-and-its-treatment.

9. Office on Women's Health, US Department of Health and Human Services, "Infertility," www.womenshealth.gov/a-z-topics/infertility.

10. Elissa Strauss, "Fertility Testing Is Big Business—But Is It Really Helping You Get Pregnant?" *Glamour*, December 28, 2017, www.glamour.com/story/is-fertility-testing-really-helping-you-get-pregnant.

11. National Partnership for Women and Families, "Study Examines Physicians' Perceptions of Fertility Risks Based on Race, Socioeconomic Status, Other Factors," *Women's Health Policy Report*, March 25, 2010, http://qualitycarenow.nationalpartnership.org/site/News2?abbr=daily3_&page=NewsArticle&id=23814.

12. Belle Boggs, "The Significance of Michelle Obama's Fertility Story," *Atlantic*, November 2018, www.theatlantic.com/family/archive/2018/11/michelle-obamas-ivf-story-means-lot-black-women/575824.

13. Ibid.

14. Heather Huhman, "4 Frustrating Facts about PCOS . . . and What They Mean for You." *HuffPost*, December 6, 2017, www.huffingtonpost.com/heather-huhman/frustrating-facts-about-pcos_b_7686030.html.

15. PCOS Foundation, "What Is PCOS?" www.pcosfoundation.org/PCOS-Education-trifold.pdf.

16. UChicagoMedicine, "Health Risks Associated with PCOS," https://www.uchicagomedicine.org/conditions-services/endocrinology-metabolic-disorders/polycystic-ovary-syndrome/pcos-risk.

17. Katie Estes, PhD, "Risk for Liver Disease Doubles in Women with Polycystic Ovary Syndrome," Endocrineweb, last updated December 21, 2017, www.endocrineweb.com/professional/pcos/risk-liver-disease-doubles-women-polycystic-ovary-syndrome.

18. M. Mansson et al., "Women with Polycystic Ovary Syndrome Are Often Depressed or Anxious—A Case Control Study," *Psychoneuroendocrinology* 33, no. 8 (September 2008): 1132–38, www.ncbi.nlm.nih.gov/pubmed/18672334.

19. Cision PR Newswire, "U.S. Senate Unanimously Passes Historic Polycystic Ovary Syndrome (PCOS) Resolution," December 28, 2017, https://www.prnewswire.com/news-releases/us-senate-unanimously-passes-historic-polycystic-ovary-syndrome-pcos-resolution-300575636.html.

20. Rana Awdish, MD, *In Shock: My Journey from Death to Recovery and the Redemptive Power of Hope* (New York: St. Martin's, 2017), 46–47.

21. Ibid., 118–19.

22. Rutgers Robert Wood Johnson Medical School, "Stop. Look. Listen! Highlights from 'To Have and to Hold: Maternal Safety and the Delivery of Safe Patient Care,'" www.rwjms.rutgers.edu/RURWJ_SSLAnmatedPDF_FIN/document.pdf.

23. Ryan Hansen, "Tara's Story," Tara Hansen Foundation, July 7, 2016, https://youtu.be/hxznMy-Y0Xg.

24. Rachel Rabkin Peachman, "What You Don't Know about Your Doctor Could Hurt You," *Consumer Reports*, April 20, 2016, www.consumerreports.org/cro/health/doctors-and-hospitals/what-you-dont-know-about-your-doctor-could-hurt-you/index.htm.

25. Harriet Ryan and Matt Hamilton, "More Than 20 Women Accused a Prominent Pasadena Obstetrician of Mistreating Them. He Denied Claims and Was Able to Continue Practicing," *Los Angeles Times*, December 9, 2018, www.latimes.com/local/lanow/la-me-huntington-doctor-misconduct-allegations-20181209-story.html.

26. Nina Martin and Renee Montagne, "Focus on Infants during Childbirth Leaves U.S. Moms in Danger," *Morning Edition*, May 12, 2017, www.npr.org/2017/05/12/527806002/focus-on-infants-during-childbirth-leaves-u-s-moms-in-danger.

27. Alison Young, "Hospitals Know How to Protect Mothers. They Just Aren't Doing It," *USA Today*, July 27, 2018, www.usatoday.com/in-depth/news/investigations/deadly-deliveries/2018/07/26/maternal-mortality-rates-preeclampsia-postpartum-hemorrhage-safety/546889002.

28. Sumathi Reddy, "A Troubling Rise in Pregnancy-Related Heart Problems," *Wall Street Journal*, August 13, 2018, www.wsj.com/articles/a-troubling-rise-in-pregnancy-related-heart-problems-1534168935.

29. Centers for Disease Control and Prevention, "Pregnancy-Related Deaths," www.cdc.gov/reproductivehealth/maternalinfanthealth/pregnancy-relatedmortality.htm.

30. Kim Brooks, "America Is Blaming Pregnant Women for Their Own Deaths," *New York Times*, November 16, 2018, www.nytimes.com/2018/11/16/opinion/sunday/maternal-mortality-rates.html.

31. Rob Haskell, "Serena Williams on Motherhood, Marriage, and Making Her Comeback," *Vogue*, January 10, 2018, www.vogue.com/article/serena-williams-vogue-cover-interview-february-2018.

32. Linda Villarosa, "Why America's Black Mothers and Babies Are in a Life-or-Death Crisis," *New York Times Magazine*, April 11, 2018, www.nytimes.com/2018/04/11/magazine/black-mothers-babies-death-maternal-mortality.html.

33. Ibid.

34. Tanya Burrwell, "Postpartum Depression and Race: What We All Should Know," Psychology Benefits Society, June 21, 2016, https://psychologybenefits.org/2016/06/21/postpartum-depression-in-women-of-color.

35. Hui Xu et al., "Cesarean Section and Risk of Postpartum Depression: A Meta-analysis," *Journal of Psychosomatic Research* 97 (June 2017): 118–26, www.jpsychores.com/article/S0022-3999(17)30052-1/fulltext.

36. Tara Haelle, "Your Biggest C-Section Risk May Be Your Hospital," *Consumer Reports*, May 10, 2018, www.consumerreports.org/c-section/biggest-c-section-risk-may-be-your-hospital.

37. Donald A. Barr, MD, PhD, "A Time to Listen," *Annals of Internal Medicine*, January 20, 2004, http://annals.org/aim/article-abstract/717100/time-listen.

38. Barbara A. Goff, MD, et al., "Ovarian Carcinoma Diagnosis," *Cancer* 89, no. 10 (November 15, 2000): 2068–75, https://onlinelibrary.wiley.com/doi/full/10.1002/1097-0142%2820001115%2989%3A10%3C2068%3A%3AAID-CNCR6%3E3.0.CO%3B2-Z.

39. Barbara A. Goff, MD, et al., "Frequency of Symptoms of Ovarian Cancer in Women Presenting to Primary Care Clinics," *Journal of the American Medical Association* 291, no. 22 (June 9, 2004): 2705–12, www.ncbi.nlm.nih.gov/pubmed/15187051.

40. Patricia Jasen, "From the 'Silent Killer' to the 'Whispering Disease': Ovarian Cancer and the Uses of Metaphor," *Medical History* 53, no. 4 (October 2009): 489–512, www.ncbi.nlm.nih.gov/pmc/articles/PMC2766137.

41. Shannon Cohn, "The Most Common Disease You've Never Heard Of," TED Talk at the University of Mississippi, March 8, 2017, www.youtube.com/watch?v=pLCeQyxVWB8.

42. Endometriosis Foundation of American, "What Is Endometriosis?" www.endofound.org/endometriosis.

43. Endometriosis Association, www.endometriosisassn.org/endo.html.

44. American College of Obstetricians and Gynecologists, Frequently Asked Questions, "Endometriosis," www.acog.org/Patients/FAQs/Endometriosis.

45. Ibid.

46. Marina Kvaskoff, PhD, "Endometriosis and Co-morbidities," http://endometriosis.org/news/research/endometriosis-and-comorbidities.

47. Cohn, "The Most Common Disease You've Never Heard Of."

48. Abby Norman, *Ask Me about My Uterus* (New York: Nation Books, 2018), 148.

49. Ibid., 256.

50. Elizabeth A. Stewart, MD, et al., "The Burden of Uterine Fibroids for African-American Women: Results of a National Survey," *Journal of Women's Health* 22, no. 10 (October 2013): 807–16, www.ncbi.nlm.nih.gov/pmc/articles/PMC3787340.

51. National Institutes of Health, US Department of Health and Human Services, "How Many People Are Affected by or At Risk of Uterine Fibroids?" www.nichd.nih.gov/health/topics/uterine/conditioninfo/people-affected.

52. US Food and Drug Administration, "Premarket Notification 510(k)," www.fda.gov/MedicalDevices/DeviceRegulationandGuidance/HowtoMarketYourDevice/PremarketSubmissions/PremarketNotification510k/default.htm.

53. Mayo Clinic, "Myomectomy," www.mayoclinic.org/tests-procedures/myomectomy/about/pac-20384710.

54. Ibid.

55. Denise Grady, "Uterine Surgical Technique Is Linked to Abnormal Growths and Cancer Spread," *New York Times*, February 6, 2014, www.nytimes.com/2014/02/07/health/uterine-surgical-technique-is-linked-to-abnormal-growths-and-cancer-spread.html.

56. "Deadly Medicine" (series), *Wall Street Journal*, November 22, 2014–December 9, 2014, www.pulitzer.org/files/2015/public-service/wsj/01wsj2015.pdf.

57. Ed Susman, "Big Concerns about Inadvertent Use of Morcellation in Previously Undiagnosed Uterine Leiomyosarcoma," *Oncology Times* 33, no. 10

(May 25, 2011): 64, 66–67, https://journals.lww.com/oncology-times/fulltext/2011/05250/Big_Concerns_about_inadvertent_Use_of_Morcellation.15.aspx.

58. M. A. Seidman et al., "Peritoneal Dissemination Complicating Morcellation of Uterine Mesenchymal Neoplasms," *PLoS One* 7, no. 11 (2012), www.ncbi.nlm.nih.gov/pubmed/23189178.

59. Sandy Hingston, "What Are the Chances?" *Boston*, March 20, 2016, www.bostonmagazine.com/health/2016/03/20/amy-reed-morcellation.

60. Matthew Bin Han Ong, "Amy Reed, Physician and Patient Who 'Moved Mountains' to End Widespread Use of Power Morcellation, Dies at 44," *Cancer Letter*, May 26, 2017, https://cancerletter.com/articles/20170526_1.

61. Ibid.

62. Denise Fulton, "VIDEO: Public Testimony Gets Heated at FDA Panel Meeting on Morcellation," *Oncology Practice*, July 11, 2014, www.mdedge.com/oncologypractice/article/84441/gynecologic-cancer/video-public-testimony-gets-heated-fda-panel.

63. US Food and Drug Administration, "Immediately in Effect Guidance Document: Product Labeling for Laparoscopic Power Morcellators," November 25, 2014, www.fda.gov/downloads/MedicalDevices/DeviceRegulationandGuidanceDocuments/UCM424123.pdf.

64. Jon Kamp and Jennifer Levitz, "Surgical Tool Gets Strongest Warning," *Wall Street Journal*, November 24, 2014, www.wsj.com/articles/fda-adds-new-warning-to-labels-for-laparoscopic-power-morcellator-1416842439.

65. Amy Martyn, "The Many Women Suing Johnson & Johnson," ConsumerAffairs, August 30, 2017, www.consumeraffairs.com/news/the-many-women-suing-johnson-johnson-083017.html.

66. American College of Obstetricians and Gynecologists, "ACOG Statement on Power Morcellation," November 24, 2014, www.acog.org/About-ACOG/News-Room/Statements/2014/ACOG-Statement-on-Power-Morcellation.

67. Denise Grady and Katie Thomas, "F.B.I. Investigates Whether Harm from Surgical Power Tool Was Ignored," *New York Times*, May 27, 2015, www.nytimes.com/2015/05/28/business/fbi-investigates-whether-harm-from-surgical-power-tool-was-ignored.html.

68. Jennifer Levitz, "Members of Congress Call on GAO to Investigate Surgical Tool," *Wall Street Journal*, August 7, 2015, www.wsj.com/articles/members-of-congress-call-on-gao-to-investigate-surgical-tool-1438978884.

69. Dr. Hooman Noorchashm, "United States Attorneys Office: Indict STORZ Executives For Criminal Negligence Causing American Deaths," *Medium*, September 28, 2017, https://medium.com/@noorchashm/united-states-attorneys-office-indict-storz-executives-for-criminal-negligence-and-homicide-437b8a276c50.

70. Matthew Bin Han Ong, "Judge Rebukes Brigham for Placing Morcellation Critic under Guard While His Wife Was in Surgery," *Cancer Letter*, November 3, 2015, https://cancerletter.com/articles/20151103_11.

71. Sheila Kaplan, "Bayer Will Stop Selling the Troubled Essure Birth Control Implants," *New York Times*, July 20, 2018, www.nytimes.com/2018/07/20/health/bayer-essure-birth-control.html.

72. Hooman Noorchashm, MD, PhD, and Amy J. Reed, MD, PhD, "Essure: Another FDA Failure to Regulate," *Philadelphia Inquirer*, October 1, 2015, www.philly.com/philly/blogs/healthcare/Essure-Another-FDA-failure-to-regulate.html.

73. US Food and Drug Administration, "Statement from FDA Commissioner Scott Gottlieb, M.D., on Manufacturer Announcement to Halt Essure Sales in the U.S.; Agency's Continued Commitment to Postmarket Review of Essure and Keeping Women Informed," July 20, 2018, www.fda.gov/NewsEvents/Newsroom/PressAnnouncements/ucm614123.htm.

74. Will Boggs, MD, "Doctors Dispute FDA's Ruling on Uterine Surgery Technique," Reuters Health News, December 8, 2015, www.reuters.com/article/us-health-uterus-fibroids/doctors-dispute-fdas-ruling-on-uterine-surgery-technique-idUSKBN0TR2TX20151208.

75. William H. Parker, MD, et al., "U.S. Food and Drug Administration's Guidance Regarding Morcellation of Leiomyomas: Well-Intentioned, But Is It Harmful for Women?" *Obstetrics & Gynecology* 127, no. 1 (January 2016): 18–22, https://journals.lww.com/greenjournal/Abstract/2016/01000/U_S_Food_and_Drug_Administration_s_Guidance.5.aspx.

76. Fulton, "Public Testimony Gets Heated at FDA Panel Meeting on Morcellation."

77. US Food and Drug Administration, "FDA Allows Marketing of First-of-Kind Tissue Containment System for Use with Certain Laparoscopic Power Morcellators in Select Patients," news release, April 7, 2016, www.fda.gov/NewsEvents/Newsroom/PressAnnouncements/ucm494650.htm.

78. Jessica Bartlett, "Doctor Who Took on Medical Manufacturers Dies," *Boston Business Journal*, May 26, 2017, www.bizjournals.com/triangle/bizwomen/news/latest-news/2017/05/doctor-who-took-on-medical-manufacturers-dies.html.

79. Michelle Llamas, "Sarah Salem-Robinson Talks about Morcellators and Complications," *Drugwatch* (podcast), August 14, 2017, https://www.drugwatch.com/podcast/sarah-salem-robinson-talks-morcellators-complications/.

80. V. B. Desai et al., "Occult Gynecologic Cancer in Women Undergoing Hysterectomy or Myomectomy for Benign Indications," *Journal of Obstetrics*

and Gynecology 131, no. 4 (April 2018): 642–51, www.ncbi.nlm.nih.gov/pubmed/29528920.

81. Comment from Stephen Hunt, MD, PhD, on citizen petition from Hooman Noorchashm, www.regulations.gov/document?D=FDA-2018-P-3843-0099.

82. US Food and Drug Administration, "Statement from FDA Commissioner Scott Gottlieb, M.D. and Jeff Shuren, M.D., Director of the Center for Devices and Radiological Health, on FDA's Updates to Medical Device Safety Action Plan to Enhance Post-market Safety," November 20, 2018, www.fda.gov/NewsEvents/Newsroom/PressAnnouncements/ucm626286.htm.

83. International Consortium of Investigative Journalists, "Medical Devices Harm Patients Worldwide as Governments Fail on Safety," *Implant Files*, November 25, 2018, www.icij.org/investigations/implant-files/medical-devices-harm-patients-worldwide-as-governments-fail-on-safety.

4. HEARTFELT

1. *The Fosters*, season 5, episode 15, "Mother's Day," aired February 13, 2018, www.tvguide.com/tvshows/the-fosters/episodes/406459.

2. Centers for Disease Control and Prevention, "Women and Heart Disease Fact Sheet," www.cdc.gov/dhdsp/data_statistics/fact_sheets/fs_women_heart.htm.

3. Go Red for Women, American Heart Association, "Heart Disease in Hispanic Women," www.goredforwomen.org/about-heart-disease/facts_about_heart_disease_in_women-sub-category/hispanic-women.

4. National Heart, Lung, and Blood Institute, National Institutes of Health, "The Heart Truth for African American Women," https://www.nhlbi.nih.gov/sites/default/files/publications/16-5066.pdf.

5. "Uncovering the Link between Emotional Stress and Heart Disease," *Harvard Heart Letter*, April 2017, www.health.harvard.edu/heart-disease-overview/uncovering-the-link-between-emotional-stress-and-heart-disease.

6. "Women 50% More Likely Than Men to Be Given Incorrect Diagnosis Following Heart Attack," *Cardiovascular News*, September 5, 2016, https://cardiovascularnews.com/women-50-more-likely-than-men-to-be-given-incorrect-diagnosis-following-heart-attack.

7. *Grey's Anatomy*, season 14, episode 11, "(Don't Fear) the Reaper," written by Elisabeth R. Finch, aired February 1, 2018, https://abc.go.com/shows/greys-anatomy/episode-guide/season-14.

8. Ibid.

9. Elisabeth R. Finch, "I Confronted the Doctor Who Missed My Cancer," *Elle*, January 5, 2016, www.elle.com/life-love/a32907/i-confronted-the-doctor-who-missed-my-cancer.

10. Center on Media and Human Development, School of Communication, Northwestern University, *Teens, Health, and Technology, A National Survey*, June 2015, https://cmhd.northwestern.edu/wp-content/uploads/2015/05/1886_1_ SOC_ConfReport_TeensHealthTech_051115.pdf.

11. Go Red for Women, American Heart Association, "About Go Red," https://www.goredforwomen.org/en/about-us.

12. American Heart Association, "Heart Attack Symptoms in Women," www. heart.org/HEARTORG/Conditions/HeartAttack/WarningSignsofaHeartAttack/ Heart-Attack-Symptoms-in-Women_UCM_436448_Article.jsp#.WmETpZM-c_ U.

13. Mayo Clinic, "Heart Disease in Women: Understand Symptoms and Risk Factors," www.mayoclinic.org/diseases-conditions/heart-disease/in-depth/heart-disease/art-20046167.

14. Rosie O'Donnell, "My Heart Attack," August 20, 2012, *Rosie.com* (blog), www.rosie.com/my-heart-attack.

15. American Heart Association, "Most Young Women Don't Recognize Heart Attack Warning Signs," *ScienceDaily*, May 11, 2007, www.sciencedaily. com/releases/2007/05/070510160957.htm.

16. Michael Greenwood, "Heart Attack Symptoms Often Misinterpreted in Younger Women," YaleNews, February 19, 2018, https://news.yale.edu/2018/ 02/19/heart-attack-symptoms-often-misinterpreted-younger-women.

17. Women Heart: The National Coalition for Women with Heart Disease, www.womenheart.org.

18. Harvard Health Publishing, Harvard Medical School "Gender Matters: Heart Disease Risk in Women," last updated March 25, 2017, www.health. harvard.edu/heart-health/gender-matters-heart-disease-risk-in-women.

19. Gayatri Devi, MD, *The Spectrum of Hope: An Optimistic and New Approach to Alzheimer's Disease and Other Dementias* (New York: Workman, 2017), 134–35.

20. Ibid.

21. University of Colorado, OB/GYN & Family Planning, "Heart Disease & Birth Control," https://obgyn.coloradowomenshealth.com/health-info/birth-control/medical-conditions-birth-control/heart-disease.

22. U.S. Department of Health and Human Services, National Institutes of Health, National Heart, Lung, and Blood Institute, "The Healthy Heart Handbook for Women," https://www.nhlbi.nih.gov/files/docs/public/heart/ hdbk_wmn.pdf.

23. George Washington University, "Women and Men with Heart Attack Symptoms Get Different Treatment from EMS," EurekAlert! December 11, 2018, www.eurekalert.org/pub_releases/2018-12/gwu-wam121118.php.

24. Nieca Goldberg, MD, *Women Are Not Small Men: Life-Saving Strategies for Preventing and Healing Heart Disease in Women* (New York: Ballantine Books, 2002).

25. Tara Parker-Pope, "Should You Choose a Female Doctor?" *New York Times*, August 14, 2018, www.nytimes.com/2018/08/14/well/doctors-male-female-women-men-heart.html.

26. Washington University in St. Louis, "Women Survive Heart Attacks Better with Women Doctors," *ScienceDaily*, August 6, 2018, www.sciencedaily.com/releases/2018/08/180806152045.htm.

27. Brad N. Greenwood et al., "Patient-Physician Gender Concordance and Increased Mortality among Female Heart Attack Patients," *Proceedings of the National Academy of Sciences* 115, no. 34 (August 21, 2018), www.pnas.org/content/115/34/8569.

28. Carolyn Thomas, *A Woman's Guide to Living with Heart Disease* (Baltimore: Johns Hopkins University Press, 2017), 1–3.

29. Ibid., 21.

30. Roni Caryn Rabin, "Is Microvascular Heart Disease a Serious Condition?" *New York Times*, September 29, 2017, www.nytimes.com/2017/09/29/well/live/is-microvascular-heart-disease-a-serious-condition.html.

31. Luke K. Kim et al., "Sex-Based Disparities in Incidence, Treatment, and Outcomes of Cardiac Arrest in the United States, 2003–2012," *Journal of the American Heart Association* 5 (2016), http://jaha.ahajournals.org/content/5/6/e003704.

32. American Heart Association, "Gender Gap Found in Cardiac Arrest Care, Outcomes," AHA/ASA Newsroom, June 22, 2016, https://newsroom.heart.org/news/gender-gap-found-in-cardiac-arrest-care-outcomes.

33. National Heart, Lung, and Blood Institute, National Institutes of Health, "What Is Long QT Syndrome?" www.nhlbi.nih.gov/health-topics/long-qt-syndrome.

34. Johns Hopkins Medicine Health Library, "Overview of Pacemakers and Implantable Cardioverter Defibrillators (ICDs)," www.hopkinsmedicine.org/healthlibrary/conditions/cardiovascular_diseases/overview_of_pacemakers_and_implantable_cardioverter_defibrillators_icds_85,P00234.

35. Derek R. MacFadden, MD, et al., "Sex Differences in Implantable Cardioverter-Defibrillator Outcomes: Findings from a Prospective Defibrillator Database," *Annals of Internal Medicine* 156, no. 3 (2012): 195–203, http://annals.org/aim/article-abstract/1033351/sex-differences-implantable-cardioverter-defibrillator-outcomes-findings-from-prospective-defibrillator.

36. Khang-Li Looi et al., "Gender Differences in the Use of Primary Prevention ICDs in New Zealand Patients with Heart Failure," *Heart Asia* 10, no. 1 (2018), www.ncbi.nlm.nih.gov/pmc/articles/PMC5786928.

37. Hadassah, Coalition for Women's Health Equity, www.hadassah.org/advocate/coalition-for-womens-health.html.

38. "Patient Advocate—Starr Mirza," Hadassah, Coalition for Women's Health Equity, May 23, 2018, https://vimeo.com/271539846.

39. American Heart Association, "A Woman's Heart Attack Causes, Symptoms May Differ from a Man's," AHA/ASA Newsroom, January 25, 2016, https://newsroom.heart.org/news/a-womans-heart-attack-causes-symptoms-may-differ-from-a-mans.

40. Will Boggs, MD, "Women Less Likely Than Men to Get Cardiac Rehab," Reuters Health News, April 27, 2016, www.reuters.com/article/us-health-women-cardiac-rehabilitation/women-less-likely-than-men-to-get-cardiac-rehab-idUSKCN0XO2HH.

41. American College of Cardiology, "Do Women-Only Cardiac Rehab Programs Benefit Female Patients?" February 3, 2016, www.acc.org/latest-in-cardiology/articles/2016/02/03/16/17/do-women-only-cardiac-rehab-programs-benefit-female-patients.

42. Mayo Clinic, "Preeclampsia," www.mayoclinic.org/diseases-conditions/preeclampsia/symptoms-causes/syc-20355745.

43. Penseé Wu et al., "Preeclampsia and Future Cardiovascular Health: A Systematic Review and Meta-analysis," *Circulation: Cardiovascular Quality and Outcomes* 10, no. 2 (February 2017), www.ahajournals.org/doi/10.1161/CIRCOUTCOMES.116.003497.

5. CHRONIC

1. Lidija Haas, "Memoirs of Disease and Disbelief," *New Yorker*, June 4 and 11, 2018, www.newyorker.com/magazine/2018/06/04/memoirs-of-disease-and-disbelief.

2. Charles W. Schmidt, MS, "Questions Persist: Environmental Factors in Autoimmune Disease," *Environmental Health Perspectives* 119, no. 6 (June 2011): A248–53, www.ncbi.nlm.nih.gov/pmc/articles/PMC3114837.

3. Margarida Azevedo, "Rise in MS and Autoimmune Disease Linked to Processed Foods," *Multiple Sclerosis News Today*, January 8, 2016, https://multiplesclerosisnewstoday.com/2016/01/08/rise-ms-autoimmune-disease-linked-processed-foods.

4. Allan Adamson, "Intense Stress and Autoimmune Diseases: Trauma May Raise Risk of Immune System Disorders," *Tech Times*, June 20, 2018, www.

techtimes.com/articles/230720/20180620/intense-stress-and-autoimmune-diseases-trauma-may-raise-risk-of-immune-system-disorders.htm.

5. American Autoimmune Related Diseases Association, "How Many Americans Have an Autoimmune Disease?" April 29, 2017, www.aarda.org/knowledge-base/many-americans-autoimmune-disease.

6. Marta Ribeiro, "10 Facts and Statistics about Autoimmune Diseases," *Scleroderma News*, October 30, 2017, https://sclerodermanews.com/2017/10/30/autoimmune-facts-statistics.

7. Liz Welch, "Autoimmune Epidemic: The Medical Experts," *SELF*, March 31, 2015, www.self.com/story/autoimmune-epidemic-doctors-working-toward-answers.

8. Sharon Worcester, "Lyme Disease Presents Differently in Men and Women," *Internal Medicine News*, March 22, 2012, www.mdedge.com/internalmedicinenews/article/49028/rheumatology/lyme-disease-presents-differently-men-and-women.

9. Emily Dwass, "The 'It's All in Your Head' Diagnosis Is Still a Danger to Women's Health," *Los Angeles Times*, July 26, 2017, www.latimes.com/opinion/op-ed/la-oe-dwass-gender-bias-medicine-20170726-story.html.

10. Mayo Clinic, "Lupus," www.mayoclinic.org/diseases-conditions/lupus/symptoms-causes/syc-20365789.

11. Stephen Feller, "Widely Used Hypertension Drugs Less Effective in Black Patients," UPI Health News, September 15, 2015, www.upi.com/Health_News/2015/09/15/Widely-used-hypertension-drugs-less-effective-in-black-patients/2411442343540.

12. Emory News Center, "African American Women Develop Lupus at a Younger Age," October 28, 2013, http://news.emory.edu/stories/2013/10/lupus_and_african_american_women/campus.html

13. Lupus Foundation of America, "Lupus Facts and Statistics," https://www.lupus.org/resources/lupus-facts-and-statistics.

14. Mayo Clinic, "Parvovirus Infection," www.mayoclinic.org/diseases-conditions/parvovirus-infection/symptoms-causes/syc-20376085.

15. Carroline P. Lobo et al., "Impact of Invalidation and Trust in Physicians on Health Outcomes in Fibromyalgia Patients," *Primary Care Companion for CNS Disorders* 16, no. 5 (October 9, 2014), www.ncbi.nlm.nih.gov/pubmed/25667809.

16. "Best Medications to Treat Fibromyalgia," *Consumer Reports,* February 2014, https://www.consumerreports.org/cro/2014/02/evaluating-prescription-drugs-used-to-treat-fibromyalgia/index.htm.

17. Emily Dwass, "Flexing against Chronic Pain," *Los Angeles Times*, May 12, 2008, http://articles.latimes.com/2008/may/12/health/he-fibro12.

18. Centers for Disease Control and Prevention, "May 12 Is ME/CFS and Fibromyalgia Awareness Day," www.cdc.gov/features/cfsawarenessday/index.html.

19. Office on Women's Health, US Department of Health and Human Services, "Chronic Fatigue Syndrome," www.womenshealth.gov/a-z-topics/chronic-fatigue-syndrome.

20. Wil S. Hylton, "The Unbreakable Laura Hillenbrand," *New York Times Magazine*, December 18, 2014, www.nytimes.com/2014/12/21/magazine/the-unbreakable-laura-hillenbrand.html.

21. Ibid.

22. Paul Costello, "Leaving Frailty Behind: A Conversation with Laura Hillenbrand," *Stanford Medicine* (summer 2016), https://stanmed.stanford.edu/2016summer/leaving-frailty-behind.html.

23. Ibid.

24. Alexandra Wolfe, "A Filmmaker's Personal Look at Chronic Fatigue Syndrome," *Wall Street Journal*, January 12, 2018, www.wsj.com/articles/a-filmmakers-personal-look-at-chronic-fatigue-syndrome-1515783784.

6. CRACKING THE CEILING

1. Changing the Face of Medicine, "Dr. Frances K. Conley," https://cfmedicine.nlm.nih.gov/physicians/biography_68.html.

2. Stanford University News Service, "Stanford Dean Discusses Resignation of Neurosurgeon Who Alleges Widespread Sexual Discrimination," June 4, 1991, https://news.stanford.edu/pr/91/910604Arc1335.html.

3. Ibid.

4. Associated Press, "Cardiology Professor at Stanford Facing Harassment Charges," *New York Times*, June 28, 1991, www.nytimes.com/1991/06/28/us/cardiology-professor-at-stanford-facing-harassment-charges.html.

5. Thomas Lee, "Marissa Mayer Feared Sexism in Medicine—So She Chose Tech Instead," *San Francisco Chronicle*, June 28, 2017, www.sfchronicle.com/business/article/Marissa-Mayer-feared-sexism-in-medicine-so-11254086.php.

6. Ashley C. Wietsma, MD, "Barriers to Success for Female Physicians in Academic Medicine," *Journal of Community Hospital Internal Medicine Perspectives* 4, no. 3 (2014), www.ncbi.nlm.nih.gov/pmc/articles/PMC4120052.

7. Ibid.

8. American Heart Association, "Women in Cardiology Mentoring Award," *Professional Heart Daily*, https://professional.heart.org/professional/MembershipCouncils/ScienticCouncils/UCM_322631_Women-in-Cardiology-Mentoring-Award.jsp.

9. Weill Cornell Medicine, "Dr. Lila Wallis, Clinical Professor at Weill Cornell, Receives 'Distinguished Women in Medicine' Award from Columbia P&S," May 17, 2002, https://news.weill.cornell.edu/news/2002/05/dr-lila-wallis-clinical-professor-at-weill-cornell-receives-distinguished-women-in-medicine-award-fr.

10. Changing the Face of Medicine, "Dr. Lila Amdurska Wallis," https://cfmedicine.nlm.nih.gov/physicians/biography_326.html.

11. Changing the Face of Medicine, "Dr. May Edward Chinn," https://cfmedicine.nlm.nih.gov/physicians/biography_61.html.

12. Crystal Emery, producer, director, writer, *Black Women in Medicine*, 2016; Boston: American Public Television.

13. Crystal R. Emery, "Black Women Are Doctors, Believe It or Not, America," *Time*, October 14, 2016, www.time.com/4532225/black-women-doctors.

14. Ibid.

15. Brittani Jackson, MD, and Brandi Jackson, MD, "Our Story," MedLikeMe, https://www.medlikeme.com/our-story.

16. Reshma Jagsi, MD, et al., "Sexual Harassment and Discrimination Experiences of Academic Medical Faculty," *Journal of the American Medical Association* 315, no. 19 (2016): 2120–21, https://jamanetwork.com/journals/jama/fullarticle/2521958.

17. Elizabeth Chuck, "#MeToo in Medicine: Women, Harassed in Hospitals and Operating Rooms, Await Reckoning," NBC News, February 20, 2018, www.nbcnews.com/storyline/sexual-misconduct/harassed-hospitals-operating-rooms-women-medicine-await-their-metoo-moment-n846031.

18. 500 Women Scientists, "NAS Report on Sexual Harassment," https://500womenscientists.org/nas-summary.

19. Alexandra Lucas et al., "Women in Cardiology: The X Factor and the Heart of Medicine," *Journal of Clinical & Experimental Cardiology* 5 (2014), www.omicsonline.org/open-access/women-in-cardiology-the-x-factor-and-the-heart-of-medicine-2155-9880-5-e134.php?aid=23887.

20. Sandra J. Lewis, MD, et al., "Changes in the Professional Lives of Cardiologists over 2 Decades," *Journal of the American College of Cardiology* 69, no. 4 (2017): 452–62, www.sciencedirect.com/science/article/pii/S0735109716371157?via%3Dihub.

21. Christopher Clarey, "For Women, a Year of Stunning Deeds and Wrenching Moments," *New York Times*, December 19, 2018, www.nytimes.com/2018/12/19/sports/for-women-a-year-of-stunning-deeds-and-wrenching-moments.html.

22. Will Hobson, "Larry Nassar, Former USA Gymnastics Doctor, Sentenced to 40–175 Years for Sex Crimes," *Washington Post*, January 24, 2018, www.washingtonpost.com/sports/olympics/larry-nassar-former-usa-gymnastics-

doctor-due-to-be-sentenced-for-sex-crimes/2018/01/24/9acc22f8-0115-11e8-8acf-ad2991367d9d_story.html.

23. Rachael Denhollander, "The Price I Paid for Taking on Larry Nassar," *New York Times*, January 26, 2018, www.nytimes.com/2018/01/26/opinion/sunday/larry-nassar-rachael-denhollander.html.

24. Matt Hamilton, Richard Winton, and Adam Elmahrek, "LAPD Begins Sweeping Criminal Probe of Former USC Gynecologist While Urging Patients to Come Forward," *Los Angeles Times*, May 29, 2018, www.latimes.com/local/lanow/la-me-usc-tyndall-lapd-20180529-story.html.

25. *Los Angeles Times* investigative team, "An Overdose, a Young Companion, Drug-Fueled Parties: The Secret Life of USC Med School Dean," *Los Angeles Times*, July 17, 2017, www.latimes.com/local/california/la-me-usc-doctor-20170717-htmistory.html.

26. Sarah Parvini et al., "USC Medical School Dean Out Amid Revelations of Sexual Harassment Claim, $135,000 Settlement with Researcher," *Los Angeles Times*, October 6, 2017, www.latimes.com/local/lanow/la-me-usc-dean-harassment-20171005-story.html.

27. Carrie Teegardin et al., "License to Betray," *Atlanta Journal & Constitution*, July 2016, http://doctors.ajc.com/doctors_sex_abuse/?ecmp=doctorssexabuse_microsite_nav.

28. Carol K. Bates, MD, et al., "It Is Time for Zero Tolerance for Sexual Harassment in Academic Medicine," *Academic Medicine* 93, no. 2 (February 2018), https://journals.lww.com/academicmedicine/Abstract/2018/02000/It_Is_Time_for_Zero_Tolerance_for_Sexual.15.aspx.

29. Alanna Vagianos, "Why Women Surgeons around the World Are Recreating This Magazine Cover," *HuffPost*, April 11, 2017, www.huffingtonpost.com/entry/women-around-the-world-re-created-this-magazine-cover-to-show-what-a-surgeon-looks-like_us_58ed0958e4b0c89f9121ef24.

30. Christina Frangou, "Surgeons (Women and Men) Say It's Time to Close Surgery's Gender Gap," *General Surgery News*, February 6, 2018, www.generalsurgerynews.com/In-the-News/Article/02-18/Surgeons-Women-and-Men-Say-It-s-Time-to-Close-Surgery-s-Gender-Gap/46919.

31. Heather Sarsons, "Interpreting Signals in the Labor Market: Evidence from Medical Referrals," Harvard University, November 28, 2017, https://scholar.harvard.edu/files/sarsons/files/sarsons_jmp.pdf.

32. Adrienne N. Bruce et al., "Perceptions of Gender-Based Discrimination during Surgical Training and Practice," *Medical Education Online* 20 (2015), www.ncbi.nlm.nih.gov/pmc/articles/PMC4317470.

33. Ibid.

34. Doximity, "New Study Reveals Significant Gaps in U.S. Doctor Compensation," April 26, 2017, www.doximity.com/press_releases/new_study_reveals_ significant_gaps_in_us_doctor_compensation.

35. "Female Gastros Still Face Pay Inequality," *Gastroenterology & Endoscopy News*, March 13, 2018, www.gastroendonews.com/In-the-News/Article/03-18/Female-Gastros-Still-Face-Pay-Inequality/47110.

36. Valerie Gleaton, "Female Gastroenterologists Make Significantly Less than Male Counterparts," ACOG Career Connection, April 5, 2018, www. healthecareers.com/acog/article/salary/female-gastroenterologists-make-significantly-less.

37. Ulrike Muench, PhD, RN, et al., "Salary Differences between Male and Female Registered Nurses in the United States," *Journal of the American Medical Association* 313, no. 2 (2015): 1265–67, https://jamanetwork.com/journals/ jama/fullarticle/2208795.

38. Ibid.

39. Eli Wolfe, "Violence against Emergency Room Staffers Seen as Increasing," FairWarning, October 3, 2018, www.fairwarning.org/2018/10/violence-emergency-rooms-workplace-physicians-nurses.

40. Nurse.org Staff Writer, "Sexual Harassment in Nursing—It's More Common Than You Think," Nurse.org, October 13, 2017, https://nurse.org/articles/ harvey-weinstein-and-harassment-against-nurses.

41. Neil Genzlinger, "William McBride, Who Warned about Thalidomide, Dies at 91," *New York Times*, July 15, 2018, www.nytimes.com/2018/07/15/ obituaries/william-mcbride-who-warned-about-thalidomide-dies-at-91.html.

42. "These Nurses Are Also Inventors," DiversityNursing.com, November 30, 2017, https://diversitynursing.com/these-nurses-are-also-inventors.

43. Julia A. Files, MD, et al., "Speaker Introductions at Internal Medicine Grand Rounds: Forms of Address Reveal Gender Bias," *Journal of Women's Health* 26, no. 5 (May 2017), www.liebertpub.com/doi/pdf/10.1089/JWH.2016. 6044.

44. Loren G. Rabinowitz, MD, "Recognizing Blind Spots—A Remedy for Gender Bias in Medicine?" *New England Journal of Medicine* 378 (2018): 2253–55, www.nejm.org/doi/full/10.1056/NEJMp1802228.

7. "THERE IS SOMEBODY SITTING HERE"

1. Mayo Clinic, "Aortic Valve Stenosis," www.mayoclinic.org/diseases-conditions/aortic-stenosis/symptoms-causes/syc-20353139.

2. Breastcancer.org, "HER2 Status," www.breastcancer.org/symptoms/ diagnosis/her2.

3. National Cancer Institute, "TAILORx Trial Finds Most Women with Early Breast Cancer Do Not Benefit from Chemotherapy," June 3, 2018, www.cancer.gov/news-events/press-releases/2018/tailorx-breast-cancer-chemotherapy.

4. Denise Grady, "Good News for Women with Breast Cancer: Many Don't Need Chemo," *New York Times*, June 3, 2018, www.nytimes.com/2018/06/03/health/breast-cancer-chemo.html.

5. Denise Grady, "Immune-Based Treatment Helps Fight Aggressive Breast Cancer, Study Finds," *New York Times*, October 20, 2018, www.nytimes.com/2018/10/20/health/breast-cancer-immunotherapy.html.

6. Rana Awdish, MD, *In Shock: My Journey from Death to Recovery and the Redemptive Power of Hope* (New York: St. Martin's, 2017), 136–37.

7. "Insider Tips to Maximize Your Doctor Visit," *Harvard Health Letter*, February 2018, www.health.harvard.edu/staying-healthy/insider-tips-to-maximize-your-doctor-visit.

8. Emily Dwass, "After Jolt of a Medical Crisis, Support Is Key as Patients Choose Path," *Los Angeles Times*, July 18, 2014, www.latimes.com/health/la-he-crisis-20140719-story.html.

9. Theresa Brown, "How to Quantify a Nurse's 'Gut Feelings,'" *New York Times*, August 9, 2018, www.nytimes.com/2018/08/09/opinion/sunday/nurses-gut-feelings-rothman.html.

10. Dana Levinson, "8 Health Issues You Had No Idea Transgender and Gender-Diverse People Are Dealing With," *Women's Health*, July 6, 2017, www.womenshealthmag.com/health/transgender-health-issues.

11. Dima Elissa et al., "The Impact of Sex and Gender on Innovation and Health Technology," *DePaul Journal of Health Care Law* 18, no. 3 (spring 2016), https://via.library.depaul.edu/cgi/viewcontent.cgi?referer=https://www.google.com/&httpsredir=1&article=1359&context=jhcl.

12. Laura Arrowsmith, "When Doctors Refuse to See Transgender Patients, the Consequences Can Be Dire," *Washington Post*, November 26, 2017, www.washingtonpost.com/national/health-science/when-doctors-refuse-to-see-transgender-patients-the-consequences-can-be-dire/2017/11/24/d063b01c-c960-11e7-8321-481fd63f174d_story.html.

13. Smathi Reddy, "With Insurers on Board, More Hospitals Offer Transgender Surgery," *Wall Street Journal*, September 26, 2016, www.wsj.com/articles/with-insurers-on-board-more-hospitals-offer-transgender-surgery-1474907475.

14. Daniel Trotta, "Transgender Patients Face Fear and Stigma in Doctor's Office," Reuters, September 14, 2016, www.reuters.com/article/us-usa-lgbt-medicine/transgender-patients-face-fear-and-stigma-in-the-doctors-office-idUSKCN11L0AJ.

15. Donald A. Barr, MD, PhD, "A Time to Listen," *Annals of Internal Medicine*, January 20, 2004, http://annals.org/aim/article-abstract/717100/time-listen.

16. Paul Costello, "Leaving Frailty Behind: A Conversation with Laura Hillenbrand," *Stanford Medicine* (summer 2016), https://stanmed.stanford.edu/2016summer/leaving-frailty-behind.html.

AFTERWORD

1. Tom Frieden, "The Delta Variant and Beyond: Learning to Live with COVID," *Wall Street Journal*, August 13, 2021, www.wsj.com/articles/the-delta-variant-and-beyond-learning-to-live-with-covid-11628866931.

2. The Sex, Gender and COVID-19 Project, https://globalhealth5050.org/the-sex-gender-and-covid-19-project/.

3. David Cox, "Why Are Women More Prone to Long COVID?" *Guardian*, June 13, 2021, www.theguardian.com/society/2021/jun/13/why-are-women-more-prone-to-long-covid.

4. Andy Slavitt, *Preventable: The Inside Story of How Leadership Failures, Politics, and Selfishness Doomed the US Coronavirus Response* (New York: St. Martin's, 2021), 46–47.

5. Alice Broster, "Why Are Women More Likely to Suffer from Long COVID, According to Studies?" *Forbes*, March 29, 2021, www.forbes.com/sites/alicebroster/2021/03/29/why-are-women-much-more-likely-to-suffer-from-long-covid-according-to-studies/?sh=1d19b7806bc8.

6. Elizabeth Chuck, "These Women's Coronavirus Symptoms Never Went Away. Their Doctors' Willingness to Help Did," NBC News, July 28, 2020, www.nbcnews.com/news/us-news/these-women-s-coronavirus-symptoms-haven-t-gone-away-doctors-n1235091.

7. Tiffany N. Ford, Sarah Reber, and Richard V. Reeves, "Race Gaps in COVID-19 Deaths Are Even Bigger Than They Appear," Brookings Institution, June 16, 2020, www.brookings.edu/blog/up-front/2020/06/16/race-gaps-in-covid-19-deaths-are-even-bigger-than-they-appear/.

8. APM Research Lab, "The Color of Coronavirus: COVID-19 Deaths by Race and Ethnicity in the US," March 5, 2021, www.apmresearchlab.org/covid/deaths-by-race.

9. Manny Fernandez, Julie Bosman, Amy Harmon, Danielle Ivory, and Mitch Smith, "The Virus Is Devastating the US, and Leaving an Uneven Toll," *New York Times*, December 9, 2020, www.nytimes.com/2020/12/04/us/covid-united-states-surge.html.

10. Karen Feldscher, "More Men Than Women Are Dying from COVID-19. Why?" Harvard T.H. Chan School of Public Health, July 31, 2020, www.hsph.

harvard.edu/news/features/more-men-than-women-are-dying-from-covid-19-why/.

11. Averi Harper, "COVID-19 Exposes Mistrust, Health Care Inequality Going Back Generations for African Americans," ABC News, April 28, 2020, https://abcnews.go.com/Health/covid-19-exposes-mistrust-health-care-inequality-back/story?id=70370949.

12. Arielle Mitropoulos and Mariya Moseley, "Beloved Brooklyn Teacher, 30, Dies of Coronavirus after She Was Twice Denied a COVID-19 Test," ABC News, April 28, 2020, https://abcnews.go.com/Health/beloved-brooklyn-teacher-30-dies-coronavirus-denied-covid/story?id=70376445.

13. Jane Spencer and Christina Jewett, "12 Months of Trauma: 3,600 US Health Workers Died in Covid's First Year," Kaiser Health News, April 8, 2021, https://khn.org/news/article/us-health-workers-deaths-covid-lost-on-the-frontline/.

14. Louis Pilla, "Nurses Suffer Heavy Toll from COVID-19," *DailyNurse*, November 17, 2020, https://dailynurse.com/nurses-suffer-heavy-toll-from-covid-19/.

15. "Lost on the Frontline," *Guardian*, April 2021, www.theguardian.com/us-news/ng-interactive/2020/aug/11/lost-on-the-frontline-covid-19-coronavirus-us-healthcare-workers-deaths-database.

16. Robert Rosseter, Nursing Fact Sheet, American Association of Colleges of Nursing, April 1, 2019, www.aacnnursing.org/news-Information/fact-sheets/nursing-fact-sheet.

17. National Nurses United, "New Report Reveals Continued Government Failure to Track and Report Data on COVID-19 Deaths of Nurses and Other Health Care Workers," March 18, 2021, www.nationalnursesunited.org/press/new-report-reveals-continued-government-failure-to-track-and-report-covid-19-deaths-of-nurses.

18. Michelle Milford Morse and Grace Anderson, "The Shadow Pandemic: How the COVID-19 Crisis Is Exacerbating Gender Inequality," United Nation Foundation, April 14, 2020, https://unfoundation.org/blog/post/shadow-pandemic-how-covid19-crisis-exacerbating-gender-inequality/.

19. Sara Reardon, "Pandemic Measures Disproportionately Harm Women's Careers," *Nature*, March 29, 2021, https://www.nature.com/articles/d41586-021-00854-x.

20. Aaron Blake, "Fox News and Trump Are Still Pushing Hydroxychloroquine. Here's What the Data Actually Shows," *Washington Post*, June 21, 2021, www.washingtonpost.com/politics/2021/06/21/hydroxycholoroquine-coronavirus-treatment-trump-allies-cant-quit/.

21. Caroline Hallemann, "Maya Harris Is More Than Kamala Harris's Sister, She's a Key Political Ally," *Town and Country*, January 20, 2021,

www.townandcountrymag.com/society/politics/a33824505/kamala-harris-sister-maya/.

22. Cary Funk and Alec Tyson, "Growing Share of Americans Say They Plan to Get a COVID-19 Vaccine—or Already Have," Pew Research Center, March 5, 2021, www.pewresearch.org/science/2021/03/05/growing-share-of-americans-say-they-plan-to-get-a-covid-19-vaccine-or-already-have/.

23. Katelyn Fossett, "The Myth about Women and the COVID-19 Vaccine That Won't Die," *Politico*, March 26, 2021, www.politico.com/newsletters/women-rule/2021/03/26/the-myth-about-women-and-the-covid-19-vaccine-that-wont-die-492263.

24. National Institutes of Health, Notice of Special Interest (NOSI) to Encourage Administrative Supplement Applications to Investigate COVID-19 Vaccination and Menstruation, May 17, 2021, https://grants.nih.gov/grants/guide/notice-files/NOT-HD-21-035.html.

25. NIH, "Item of Interest: NIH Funds Studies to Assess Potential Effects of COVID-19 Vaccination on Menstruation," August 30, 2021, www.nichd.nih.gov/newsroom/news/083021-COVID-19-vaccination-menstruation.

26. American Medical Women's Association, www.amwa-doc.org/amwa102/saralyn-mark-md/.

27. Jeanette Beebe, "Should COVID-19 Vaccines Be Adjusted for Women?" *NextAvenue*, May 27, 2021, www.nextavenue.org/covid-vaccine-women-side-effects/.

28. Ibid.

29. Emer Brady, Mathias Wullum Nielsen, Jens Peter Anderson, and Sabine Oertelt-Prigione, "Lack of Consideration of Sex and Gender in COVID-19 Clinical Studies," *Nature Communications*, July 6, 2021, www.nature.com/articles/s41467-021-24265-8.

30. American College of Obstetricians and Gynecologists, "ACOG and SMFM Recommend COVID-19 Vaccination for Pregnant Individuals," July 30, 2021, www.acog.org/news/news-releases/2021/07/acog-smfm-recommend-covid-19-vaccination-for-pregnant-individuals.

31. National Institutes of Health, "NIH Begins Study of COVID-19 Vaccination during Pregnancy and Postpartum," June 23, 2021, www.nih.gov/news-events/news-releases/nih-begins-study-covid-19-vaccination-during-pregnancy-postpartum.

32. Yamiche Alcindor, Rachel Wellford, Bria Lloyd, and Lizz Bolaji, "With a History of Abuse in American Medicine, Black Patients Struggle for Equal Access," *PBS NewsHour*, February 24, 2021, www.pbs.org/newshour/show/with-a-history-of-abuse-in-american-medicine-black-patients-struggle-for-equal-access.

33. Kelly Bilodeau, "Migraines Linked to High Blood Pressure after Menopause," *Harvard Women's Health Watch*, August 1, 2021, www.health.harvard. edu/womens-health/migraines-linked-to-high-blood-pressure-after-menopause.

34. Sumathi Reddy, "The Surprising Good News on How Menopause Changes Your Brain," *Wall Street Journal*, June 14, 2021, www.wsj.com/ articles/the-surprising-good-news-on-how-menopause-changes-your-brain-11623698003.

35. Jen Gunter, "Women Can Have a Better Menopause. Here's How," *New York Times*, May 25, 2021, www.nytimes.com/2021/05/25/opinion/feminist-menopause.html.

36. Nick Mulcahy, "FDA Warns Again about Robotic Mastectomy, Breaks New Ground," *Medscape Medical News*, August 20, 2021, www.medscape.com/ viewarticle/957002?src=wnl_newsalrt_210820_MSCPEDIT&uac=400526DT& impID=3583111&faf=1#vp_1.

37. Jaime Dunaway, "Netflix Documentary 'The Bleeding Edge' Features Story of Arkansan's Complications after Surgery," *Arkansas Democrat Gazette*, August 3, 2018, www.arkansasonline.com/news/2018/aug/03/netflix-documentary-examining-medical-device-indus/.

38. Katherine Sanderson, "Why Sports Concussions Are Worse for Women," *Nature*, August 3, 2021, www.nature.com/articles/d41586-021-02089-2.

39. Harvey S. Levin, Nancy R. Temkin, and Jason Barber, "Association of Sex and Age with Mild Traumatic Brain Injury-Related Symptoms: A TRACK-TBI Study," *JAMA Network Open*, April 6, 2021, https://jamanetwork.com/ journals/jamanetworkopen/fullarticle/2778183.

40. Emily Paulsen, "Recognizing, Addressing Unintended Gender Bias in Patient Care," *Practice Management*, January 14, 2020, https://physicians. dukehealth.org/articles/recognizing-addressing-unintended-gender-bias-patient-care.

41. Sarah Ramey, *The Lady's Handbook for Her Mysterious Illness: A Memoir* (New York: Anchor, 2020), chap. 2.

42. Pam Kragen, "Escondido Cancer Survivor, 87, Passes 1,000 Mark in Breast-knitting Campaign," *San Diego Union-Tribune*, September 9, 2020, www.sandiegouniontribune.com/communities/north-county/escondido/story/ 2020-09-09/escondido-cancer-survivor-87-passes-1-000-mark-in-breast-knitting-campaign.

43. Maya Trabulsi, "These Tight-knit Retirees Are Helping Breast Cancer Survivors Feel Like 'Boobless Wonders,'" *PBS NewsHour*, July 26, 2021, www. pbs.org/newshour/show/these-tight-knit-retirees-are-helping-breast-cancer-survivors-feel-like-boobless-wonders.

SELECTED BIBLIOGRAPHY

BOOKS

Awdish, Rana, MD. *In Shock: My Journey from Death to Recovery and the Redemptive Power of Hope*. New York: St. Martin's, 2017.

Devi, Gayatri, MD. *The Spectrum of Hope: An Optimistic and New Approach to Alzheimer's Disease and Other Dementias*. New York: Workman, 2017.

Dusenbery, Maya. *Doing Harm: The Truth about How Bad Medicine and Lazy Science Leave Women Dismissed, Misdiagnosed, and Sick*. New York: HarperOne, 2018.

Groopman, Jerome, MD. *How Doctors Think*. Boston: Houghton Mifflin, 2007.

Katkin, Elizabeth. *Conceivability*. New York: Simon & Schuster, 2018.

Norman, Abby. *Ask Me about My Uterus: A Quest to Make Doctors Believe in Women's Pain*. New York: Nation Books, 2018.

Steinbaum, Suzanne, OD. *Dr. Suzanne Steinbaum's Heart Book: Every Woman's Guide to a Heart-Healthy Life*. New York: Penguin, 2013.

Stern, Scott W. *The Trials of Nina McCall: Sex, Surveillance, and the Decades-Long Government Plan to Imprison "Promiscuous" Women*. Boston: Beacon, 2018.

Thomas, Carolyn. *A Woman's Guide to Living with Heart Disease*. Baltimore: Johns Hopkins University Press, 2017.

NEWSPAPERS AND MAGAZINES

"Deadly Medicine" (Series). *Wall Street Journal*, November 22–December 9, 2014. www.pulitzer.org/files/2015/public-service/wsj/01wsj2015.pdf.

Hamilton, Matt, Richard Winton, and Adam Elmahrek. "LAPD Begins Sweeping Criminal Probe of Former USC Gynecologist While Urging Patients to Come Forward." *Los Angeles Times*, May 29, 2018. www.latimes.com/local/lanow/la-me-usc-tyndall-lapd-20180529-story.html.

Hingston, Sandy. "What Are the Chances?" *Boston*, March 20, 2016. www.bostonmagazine.com/health/2016/03/20/amy-reed-morcellation.

Kolata, Gina. "For Many Strokes, There's an Effective Treatment. Why Aren't Some Doctors Offering It?" *New York Times*, March 26, 2018. www.nytimes.com/2018/03/26/health/stroke-clot-buster.html.

Peachman, Rachel Rabkin. "What You Don't Know about Your Doctor Could Hurt You." *Consumer Reports*, April 20, 2016. www.consumerreports.org/cro/health/doctors-and-hospitals/what-you-dont-know-about-your-doctor-could-hurt-you/index.htm.

Pringle, Paul, Harriet Ryan, Adam Elmahrek, Matt Hamilton, and Sarah Parvini. "An Overdose, a Young Companion, Drug-Fueled Parties: The Secret Life of USC Med School Dean." *Los Angeles Times*, July 17, 2017. www.latimes.com/local/california/la-me-usc-doctor-20170717-htmistory.html.

Teegardin, Carrie, Danny Robbins, Jeff Ernsthausen, and Ariel Hart. "License to Betray." *Atlanta Journal & Constitution*, July 2016. http://doctors.ajc.com/doctors_sex_abuse/?ecmp=doctorssexabuse_microsite_nav.

Villarosa, Linda. "Why America's Black Mothers and Babies Are in a Life-or-Death Crisis." *New York Times Magazine*, April 11, 2018. www.nytimes.com/2018/04/11/magazine/black-mothers-babies-death-maternal-mortality.html.

Wolfe, Alexandra. "A Filmmaker's Personal Look at Chronic Fatigue Syndrome." *Wall Street Journal*, January 12, 2018. www.wsj.com/articles/a-filmmakers-personal-look-at-chronic-fatigue-syndrome-1515783784.

VIDEOS, FILMS, TV SHOWS, TED TALKS

Cohn, Shannon. "The Most Common Disease You've Never Heard Of." TED Talk, March 8, 2017. www.youtube.com/watch?v=pLCeQyxVWB8.

Dick, Kirby, and Amy Ziering. *The Bleeding Edge*. www.netflix.com/watch/80170862?trackId=14277281&tctx=0%2C0%2Cb3640b88-fd55-4665-b28c-c4205e11b1b6-984896682%2C%2C.

Finch, Elisabeth R. "(Don't Fear) the Reaper." *Grey's Anatomy*, season 14, February 1, 2018. https://abc.go.com/shows/greys-anatomy/episode-guide/season-14.

Hansen, Ryan. "Tara's Story." Tara Hansen Foundation, July 7, 2016. https://youtu.be/hxznMy-Y0Xg.

Johnson, Paula, MD. "When Does Medicine Leave Women Behind?" TED Talk, February 10, 2017. www.npr.org/2017/02/10/514153036/when-does-medicine-leave-women-behind.

"Sex Differences Research: Expert Commentary by Dr. Kathryn Sandberg." Georgetown University Medical Center. https://vimeo.com/36092826.

"Sex Matters: Drugs Can Affect Sexes Differently." *60 Minutes*, February 9, 2014. www.cbsnews.com/news/sex-matters-drugs-can-affect-sexes-differently.

ACKNOWLEDGMENTS

I am forever grateful to the women who shared their difficult medical journeys with me. I enormously admire and appreciate their courage and insights. Many of these women spent hours talking with me, even while dealing with ongoing medical problems. Their help and encouragement were great acts of generosity.

I also want to thank the doctors, nurses, scientists, researchers, and advocates who took time out of their busy schedules to guide me through some of the complicated issues surrounding women's health. These experts opened my eyes to the challenges women still face in medical research and clinical care.

A warm thank-you to my agent, Dana Newman, who believed in this project from the beginning and whose efforts made it a reality. I especially appreciated that Dana brought the proposal to Suzanne Staszak-Silva, who became my editor at Rowman & Littlefield. I have enjoyed working with Suzanne and know that her fine editing skills guided and greatly improved the book.

A very special thank-you to my husband, Stuart Silverstein. Not only is he an amazing partner and friend, he's also a wonderful journalist. He carefully read every word of the manuscript, making thoughtful observations and suggestions.

Finally, some words of praise for all the hardworking journalists whose investigations into women's healthcare taught me so much. These are frightening times for members of the press, especially in a hostile climate created when former President Trump maligned journalists as "enemies of the people." As my footnotes show, I relied heavily on groundbreaking reporting from many publications, especially the *New York Times*, the *Wall Street Journal*, and the *Los Angeles Times*. Often, an article by a journalist was the first step in revealing an injustice being done to women struggling to become well.

INDEX

ABOUT THE AUTHOR

Emily Dwass has written about health, food, and cultural issues for numerous publications, including the *New York Times*, the *Los Angeles Times*, *LA Weekly*, and the *Chicago Tribune*. She also has written television and movie scripts for the entertainment industry.